PEDIATRICS - LABORATORY AND CLINICAL RESEARCH

NEONATAL CARE

NEW RESEARCH

PEDIATRICS - LABORATORY AND CLINICAL RESEARCH

Additional books in this series can be found on Nova's website under the Series tab.

Additional e-books in this series can be found on Nova's website under the e-book tab.

PEDIATRICS - LABORATORY AND CLINICAL RESEARCH

NEONATAL CARE

NEW RESEARCH

FABIAN KOUBEK
AND
JUNICA LINSER
EDITORS

NOVINKA

New York

For permission to use material from this book please contact us:
Telephone 631-231-7269; Fax 631-231-8175
Web Site: http://www.novapublishers.com

Additional color graphics may be available in the e-book version of this book.

Library of Congress Cataloging-in-Publication Data

Library of Congress Control Number: 2013935081

ISBN: 978-1-62618-454-1

Published by Nova Science Publishers, Inc. † New York

CONTENTS

PREFACE

In this book, the authors present new research in the study of neonatal care. Topics discussed include the effects of maternal stress and intrauterine environmental factors on fetal behavior and central brain processes related to cognition, memory and habituation; phosphodieterases and their inhibitors in some respiratory system disorders; glucocorticoids in meconium aspiration syndrome and the possible benefits versus the risks of treatment; and the evidence linking hyperbilirubinemia to auditory neuropathy and prelingual deafness.

Chapter 1 - Several studies conducted on human beings and animals demonstrate that prenatal stress generates alterations which can be observed since birth, and which last up to adulthood. The hypothalamic-pituitary-adrenal axis (HPA) is highly sensitive to programming during development it has been suggested that the fetal programming of the HPA axis is associated with the development of cardiovascular diseases, resistance to insulin, and diabetes in adult life. Between the HPA axis and immune-inflammatory responses, a negative feedback is established. The psychoneuroendocrine pathways involve the transplacental passage of maternal glucocorticoids in order to influence directly on fetal growth and brain development. Several studies suggest that negative emotions during pregnancy generate adverse effects on the cognitive, behavioural and emotional development of the descendants.

The present work explores the role of nitric oxide and neurotrophins in the hippocampus, prefrontal cortex and cerebellum, key structures to learning and memory processes. Maternal stress and intrauterine environmental factors have a significant influence on fetal behaviour, as well as on central brain processes related with cognition, memory and habituation.

Chapter 2 – Phosphodiesterases (PDEs) represent a super-family of 11 classes of metalophosphohydrolases with ubiquitous occurrence and diverse effect. Their role in different tissues, e.g. smooth muscle, immune cells, as well as in various pathological conditions, e.g. inflammation, cough, airway hyperresponsiveness, pulmonary hypertension suggests a potential use of their inhibitors in respective therapeutic approach. In this chapter, physiological and pathophysiological roles of PDEs are reviewed with possible pharmacological modulation of their activity. Classification and pharmacological characteristics of non-selective and selective PDE inhibitors are described more in detail, e.g. mechanism of action, pharmacokinetics, and adverse effects. Special attention is drawn on use of PDE inhibitors in respiratory and inflammatory disorders, like airway hyperresponsiveness and meconium aspiration syndrome, where original experimental results are confronted with published preclinical and clinical data.

Chapter 3 – Glucocorticoids possess a lot of pharmacological properties useful in the treatment of various diseases. In meconium aspiration syndrome (MAS), a serious neonatal disease with complex pathophysiology, glucocorticoids have been administered in experimental and clinical studies with more or less success according to design of the study, type of glucocorticoid derivative, dose and mode of delivery. Nevertheless, despite growing information on positive effects of glucocorticoid treatment on the lung edema, inflammation and pulmonary vasoconstriction, many questions have not been answered yet, e.g. on possible side effects of the treatment. To consider objectively the positives and negatives of the glucocorticoid administration in MAS, this chapter reviews the pathomechanims of MAS, mechanisms of action of glucocorticoids, as well as effects of various glucocorticoids delivered in experimental models and in newborns with MAS.

Chapter 4 – Among risk factors for sensory neural hearing loss (SNHL), hyperbilirubinemia, a clinical-laboratoristic condition characterized by an excess of bilirubin in the blood, can play an important role in the development of deafness. Newborns are particularly susceptible to suffer from this pathology because of the great amount of bilirubin produced from the red cell turnover combined with the immaturity of enzymatic systems involved in bilirubin excretion.

Researchers suggested that the pathogenetic mechanism responsible of the hearing impairment consists in the deposition of bilirubin in the cochlear nuclei and in the auditory pathways. This condition occurs more frequently when total serum bilirubin exceeds 20-25 mg/dl and the unconjugated bilirubin in excess can overcome the Blood-Brain-Barrier (BBB) performing a neurotoxic action.

The main causes of hyperbilirubinemia are Rh and ABO maternal-fetal incompatibility, red cells' morphologic (as spherocytosis and elliptocytosis) and enzymatic (Glucose-6-phosphate dehydrogenase deficiency, Crigler-Najjar' syndrome, Gilbert' syndrome) defects.

Literature data is full of studies that investigate the role of hyperbilirubinemia in the development of SNHL trying to establish a total serum bilirubin (TSB) cut-off above whom newborns can be considered at high SNHL risk; nevertheless, a clear bilirubin threshold has not been defined yet. Surely, as recommended by the Joint Committee on infant hearing (JCIH) in its Position Statement of 2007, all jaundiced newborns requiring exchange transfusion should be assessed to early identify the presence of an hearing impairment.

Recent studies conducted through audiometry, otoacoustic emissions (OAEs) and auditory brainstem response (ABR), reported, in patients who suffered from hyperbilirubinemia, the presence of a cochlear and retrochlear, mainly bilateral, hearing loss with an audiometric pattern characterized by an involvement of the high frequencies.

Furthermore, among SNHL newborns who suffered from hyperbilirubinemia, it is more probable to observe a particular audiologic disease called "auditory neuropathy spectrum disorder" (ANSD), often misunderstood because of its characteristic audiologic profile (present OAEs, not recordable ABR, absence of the acoustic reflexes) that results from a damage of the cochlear inner hair cells, their synapses with the cochlear nerve or the cochlear nerve itself but with the preservation of the outer hair cells.

In: Neonatal Care: New Research
Editors: F. Koubek and J. Linser
ISBN: 978-1-62618-454-1

Chapter 1

EFFECTS OF MATERNAL STRESS ON NITRIC OXIDE AND NEUROTROPHINS IN OFFSPRING´S BRAIN

Damian G. Maur, Berenice Burdet, Joana E. Pivoz-Avedikian, María R. Larreche-Calahorrano and María A. Zorrilla-Zubilete*

Department of Pharmacology, School of Medicine,
University of Buenos Aires, Center of Pharmacological
and Botanical Studies CEFYBO-CONICET-UBA, Argentina

ABSTRACT

Several studies conducted on human beings and animals demonstrate that prenatal stress generates alterations which can be observed since birth, and which last up to adulthood. The hypothalamic-pituitary-adrenal axis (HPA) is highly sensitive to programming during development it has been suggested that the fetal programming of the HPA axis is associated

---

* Corresponding author: María A. Zorrilla-Zubilete, Department of Pharmacology, School of Medicine, University of Buenos Aires (UBA) and Center of Pharmacological and Botanical Studies (CEFYBO-CONICET) Argentina. Paraguay 2155 15°, zip code 1121, CABA, Buenos Aires, Argentina. Phone: ++54 11 5950 9500 ext. 2206; Fax: ++54 11 4508 3733, e-mail: mariazorrillaz@gmail.com.

with the development of cardiovascular diseases, resistance to insulin, and diabetes in adult life. Between the HPA axis and immune-inflammatory responses, a negative feedback is established. The psychoneuroendocrine pathways involve the transplacental passage of maternal glucocorticoids in order to influence directly on fetal growth and brain development. Several studies suggest that negative emotions during pregnancy generate adverse effects on the cognitive, behavioural and emotional development of the descendants.

The present work explores the role of nitric oxide and neurotrophins in the hippocampus, prefrontal cortex and cerebellum, key structures to learning and memory processes.

Maternal stress and intrauterine environmental factors have a significant influence on fetal behaviour, as well as on central brain processes related with cognition, memory and habituation.

Keywords: Maternal stress- nitric oxide – neurotrophins – central nervous system

INTRODUCTION

Stress is defined as any situation capable of perturbing physiological or psychological homeostasis. Exposure to adverse situations affects an important number of aspects of our daily life.

The stress response is thus referred to as “allostasis”, meaning “maintaining stability through change” (McEwen, 1998). This stress response is adaptive if it is transitory and shut off quickly with the help of feedback loops. However, in the long run, the suppression of anabolic processes, the depletion of energy stores and the suppression of the immune system can be devastating for the organism. Prolonged and/or uncontrollable sources of stress lead the organism to lose its resistance and to enter a phase of exhaustion (Sapolsky, 1992, Korte et al., 2005).

This process has been called “allostatic load”, and refers to the price the tissue or organ pays for an inefficiently managed allostatic response; more precisely, allostatic load refers to the “cost” of adaptation (McEwen, 2007). Although the stress response is a necessary survival mechanism, prolonged stress can have several negative repercussions, ranging from impairments in learning and memory to enhanced neuronal cell death (McEwen, 1999).

PRENATAL STRESS

The prenatal period is critical for the development of the nervous and immune systems. Exposure to adverse events early in life may profoundly affect brain development, leading to long-lasting effects on neuronal structure and behaviour and playing a role in the etiology of mood and anxiety disorders (de Lima et al., 2011). During this stage animals are vulnerable to factors, such as maternal stress, that can disrupt homeostasis and therefore affect development. Recent research in humans has related psychosocial work stress during pregnancy to postnatal consequences, namely the decrease in birth weight and gestational time (Lee et al., 2011). Moreover, animal studies and preliminary human studies have linked prenatal stress (PS) with alterations in development and behavioural disorders, and suggest that the effects of PS can persist long after birth (Vallee et al., 1997; Zuena et al., 2008). In fact, prenatal stress can have long lasting effects on the offspring immune system and in neurocognitive functions (Ruiz and Avant, 2005). Many studies have associated different models of PS with deficits in offspring´s development. These studies suggest that PS could predispose rats to behavioural abnormalities such as increased anxiety, greater tendency to drug addiction and depressive-like behaviour (Weinstock, 2001; Maccari et al., 2003; Mueller and Bale, 2006; Vallee et al., 1997). There has also been reported an alteration in circadian rhythms (Van Reeth et al., 1998). Behavioural studies have shown that PS offspring exhibit increased exploratory behaviour and increased locomotor activity (Vallee et al., 1997, Van den Hove et al.,2005) as well as impairments in learning and memory performance (Wu et al., 2007; Maur et al., 2012). Deficits in social behaviour are found in several neuro-psychiatric disorders with a presumed developmental origin (Patin et al., 2005).

HIPPOCAMPUS

The hippocampus is part of the limbic system. It is a structure derived from the cerebral cortex, phylogenetically old with simple and ordered structure. It is an structure of supreme interest, since it is involved in the formation of various types of memory, is a region of neurogenesis in adulthood and is linked to many other brain regions, serving an integrative function. The hippocampus consists of layers of cells morphologically and / or functionally differentiated: dentate gyrus, CA_1, CA_2, CA_3. This three sinaptic circuit receives input from the entorhinal cortex (integrative multimodal sensory) and has efferents projecting to the entorhinal cortex, the subiculum and other subcortical structures. It also connects to the hypothalamus and the suprachiasmatic nucleus. Among the neurotransmitters that are involved in this network are glutamate (mainly), GABA, ACh, DA, 5-HT, NA, neuropeptides and endocannabinoids. The hippocampus has adrenal steroid hormone receptors such as mineralocorticoid receptor (MR) and glucocorticoid receptor (GR), and gonadal and thyroid hormone receptor. Furthermore, the neurotrophins NGF and BDNF are abundant. The hippocampus develops *in utero*, but in rodents, it continues to develop postnatally. The sequence of brain development in rodents and humans is similar, however the rodent brain development at birth is equivalent in degree of progress, to the human development in the second trimester of pregnancy (Weinstock 2001). The development of CA_1 and CA_3 regions of the hippocampus in rodents occurs mainly during the third week of pregnancy, which is approximately equivalent to the early second trimester of pregnancy in humans. The peak of neurogenesís in the brain of rats and mice were is given at embryonic day 20 and 21 (Erecinska M 2004). However, the highest rate of brain maturation in mice and rats occurs postnatally, and at birth the brain has not yet completed its maturation (Erecinska M 2004).

HIPPOCAMPUS AND STRESS

Different hippocampal systems are involved in the stress response. At first the answer involves the release of NA, 5-HT and DA, and neuropeptides, such as CRH (Joels 2009). Secondly, there is switch to mechanisms triggered by glucocorticoids. In the nervous system, glucocorticoids act via two receptors: the MR and GR. The hippocampus has large amounts of glucocorticoid receptors (both GR and MR) but MR has more affinity for its ligand than GR (Mitchell JB, 1990, Maccari S 1995). Thus, when plasma concentrations of glucocorticoids (GC) are normal, MR receptors are occupied, while the GR are commonly occupied by increased GC plasma concentrations due to factors such as stress. Once activated, the receptors are translocated to the nucleus where they regulate the expression of genes and can affect the systems mentioned above, modifying the excitability of the neurons. The GR receptor activation increases the influx of Ca^{2+}, leading the cell to conditions of excitotoxicity (Chameau 2007). Furthermore, high GC plasma concentrations affect neuronal viability (Sapolsky 1986), and sustained high concentrations lead to the degeneration of hippocampal neurons (Uno et al. 1989).

The hippocampus exerts a negative feedback on the HPA axis. In rats, 50% ablation of hippocampus led to hippocampal corticosterone hypersecretion against stress (Sapolsky 1984).

In turn, stress affects the number of hippocampal GC receptors, and therefore has an effect on the HPA axis negative feedback. This was found in various models and various laboratory animals, such as rats (Maccari 1995, Zhe 2008), guinea pigs (Kapoor 2008), monkeys (Patel 2008) and birds (Hodgson 2007).

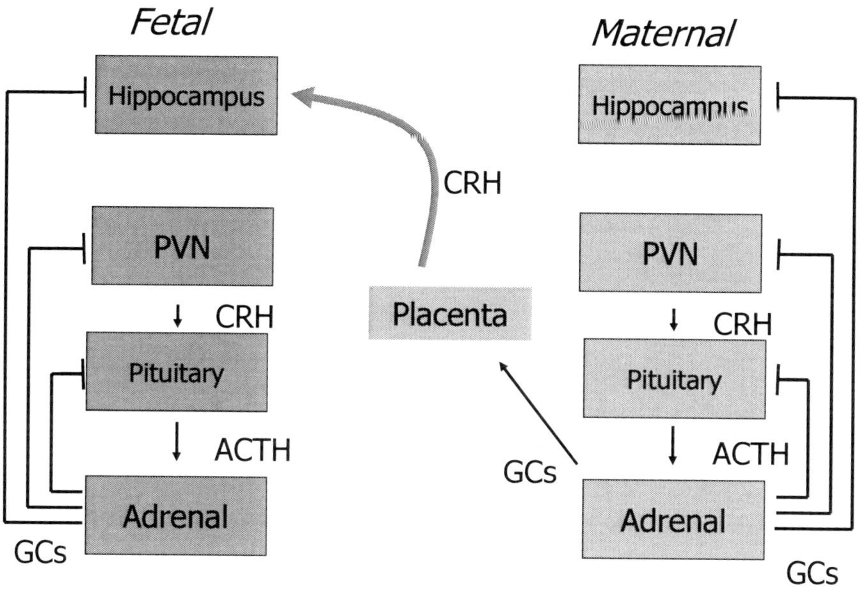

Figure 1. Interaction between maternal and fetal HPA axis.

Moreover, chronic stress induces hippocampal volume reduction (Lee 2009), a memory impediment (Palumbo et al., 2007), decreases in Long Term Potentiation (LTP) in the hippocampus (Zheng 2004) increases in glutamate hippocampal levels and decreases in GABA (Cui 2009) and BDNF expression (Li, 2009).

The decreased expression of MR/GR receptors, and the consequent increase in plasma glucocorticoids in PS animals has also been documented (Kapoor 2008, Maccari 1995). Other hippocampal alterations induced by prenatal stress are decreased neurogenesis (Lemaire 2000), reduction of LTP reduced accompanied by a reduction of NR1 and NR2B subunits of NMDA type glutamate receptor in the postsinapsis (Son 2006), a decrease in the number of GABA receptors (Fride 1985), a decrease of serotonin 5-HT1A receptor (Van den Hove et al., 2006), a decreased expression of the PKCβ1 (Wu 2007), an increase in the NA turnover (Huttunen 1971), and altered levels of metabolites of DA and 5-HT (Bowman et al. 2004).

Van den Hove et al., 2012 examined the enduring effects of PS exposure on gene expression profiles within the hippocampus and frontal cortex (FC) of adult male and female Sprague-Dawley rats. PS resulted in an increased anxiety and depression-related behaviour particularly in males. Female offspring seemed resilient to PS exposure. Moreover, PS altered the expression of numerous genes in the hippocampus and FC in a sex-specific manner.

CEREBELLUM

The cerebellum (CE), which has traditionally been related to motor functions, is currently being redefined as a structure with a much broader functionality. Human and animal research models have involved the cerebellum in cognitive functions, such as attention, perception, language and particularly working memory and spatial orientation. Animal models of cerebellar injuries of genetic origin or artificially induced, have demonstrated the role of the cerebellum in spatial orientation (Martin et al., 2003; 2004). It has also been suggested that the cerebellum is involved in emotional behaviour and motivation, the latter evaluated as motivation to explore new environments in animals in which cerebellar Purkinje and granular cells were injured (Caston et al., 1998). The studies of Bobeé et al., 2000 describe the role of the cerebellum in spatial cognition, suggesting that the cerebellar vermis is involved in motor control, attentional capabilities, territory discrimination and emotional behaviour. Passot et al., 2012 have recently shown that cerebellar deficits may impact on the exploration-exploitation balance during spatial navigation. Prenatal Stress can produce long lasting changes in cerebellar granule cell layer structure and function, such as a decrease in the number of synapses (Ulupinar and Yucel, 2005). It has been suggested therefore that stress critically affects the development of neural communications and the establishment of networks (Ulupinar and Yucel, 2005; Ulupinar et al., 2006). Maur et al., 2012 showed deficiencies in spatial memory in adult animals which were correlated with alterations in nitric oxide levels in the cerebellum of prenatally stressed rats. In this study, results show that prenatal stress exposure induced long-lasting impairments in spatial memory performance. These impairments were observed in PS adult animals, 90 days post prenatal stress and without another exposure to stress during adult life. Thus, the offspring from stressed mothers showed a higher quantity of errors, along with longer total time in the spatial memory test. In the territory discrimination test it was found that, while C animals spent more time in the unknown compartment, showing an innate preference for novelty, as expected (Poltirev et al., 1996), PS rats did not show a preference for either the known or the unknown one. This could suggest that PS rats have increased anxiety and therefore show an aversion to a novel environment. On the other hand, the results found by them might implicate that PS rats could not differentiate the two compartments.

NITRIC OXIDE

Nitric Oxide (NO) is the main product of the reaction catalyzed by nitric oxide synthase (NOS) that converts L-arginine to L-citrulline (Moncada and Higgs, 1993). The family of NOS, the enzymes that produce NO, consists of two different classes: constitutive and inducible isoforms (Dawson and Snyder 1994; Marletta 1994). Neuronal NOS (nNOS) and endothelial NOS (eNOS) are constitutive (cNOS) isoforms dependent on the transient influx of Ca2+ to activate calmodulin, which binds to the isoform to elicit enzyme activity. The inducible NOS (iNOS) is permanently bound to calmodulin, so it is not regulated by calcium concentration (Nathan and Xie, 1994) but is regulated transcriptionally (Nathan and Xie 1994; Di Monte et al. 1997). NOS is abundant in brain tissue (Marletta 1994; Araki et al. 1999; Muramatsu et al. 2003), nNOS primarily being expressed in neurons, eNOS in pyramidal cells and endothelial cells and iNOS in astrocytes, microglia, and inflammatory cells (Moncada et al. 1991).

NOS can be phosphorylated by different kinases, including protein kinase C (PKC), cyclic AMP-dependent protein kinase A, calcium-calmodulin-dependent protein kinase and cyclic GMP-dependent protein kinase (Nakane et al. 1991; Bredt et al. 1992; Dinerman et al. 1994). Phosphorylation of NOS has been shown to either stimulate (Nakane et al. 1991) or inhibit (Bredt et al. 1992; Dinerman et al. 1994) NOS activity in vitro. NO plays an important role in the control of neural activity by diffusing into neurons and participates in learning and memory processes (Chen et al. 1997). It has been demonstrated that NO plays an important role in LTP in hippocampus (Hawkins et al., 1998) and Long Term Depression (LTD) in cerebellum (Lev-Ram et al., 1997). NOS-containing neurons are found in many brain loci, including the cerebral cortex, cerebellum, hippocampus and hypothalamus. A high concentration of nNOS is present in cerebellar neurons, particularly in basket and granule cells and the pattern of localization provides a cellular basis for the involvement of NOS activity in the deleterious effects of different noxa on cerebellar function (Coyle and Puttfarken, 1993; Dawson and Dawson, 1996; Ikeda et al. 2001). NO has emerged as a key endogenous modulator of neuronal function. NO is an important brain messenger released upon activation of the glutamate N-methyl-D-aspartate (NMDA) receptor and the subsequent Ca2+-dependent activation of nNOS (Kiss and Vizi, 2001). Moreover, this molecule also has important neuromodulatory roles as a retrograde intracellular messenger mediating cell-to-cell interactions in the brain including cell-mediated immune system, cerebral smooth muscle relaxation, inhibition of platelet aggregation, synaptic plasticity and more complex processes like learning (Bredt and Snyder 1994; Schulz et al. 1995). A number of experimental studies have also demonstrated that NO and NO donors can enhance the basal release of several neurotransmitters in the mammalian brain, including dopamine, glutamate, and acetylcholine (Lonart and Johanson 1992; Nathan and Xie 1994).

The production of NO might lead to either toxicity or neuroprotection depending on the level of NO, the location of NO production, the extent of oxidative stress and the type of neurodegenerative process. It has been found that NO has both pro-oxidant and anti-oxidant actions (Lipton et al.,1993; Wink et al.,1999). Miranda et al. (2000) suggests that NO directly acts as an antioxidant. Thus, in mammalians cells, NO protects against cellular injury caused by H_2O_2, XO and alkylhydroperoxides. This protective effect is mediated by small fluxes of NO on the order of 1–2 nmol/L. This is consistent with the fact that NO terminates lipid peroxidation reactions and suggests that the production of NO is a major protective mechanism against oxidative stress *in vivo*. In fact, it was demonstrated, in vitro as well as in vivo, that during brain insult NO might be part of the physiological response to injury (Khaldi et al. 2002). In general, it is accepted that a normal pathophysiological response of the damaged tissue may involve controlled NO production and the inhibition of this response may interfere with the normal repair process. Nevertheless, it has been suggested that a high production of NO after the induction of iNOS expression participates in neurodestructive events either via formation of the toxic species peroxynitrite as a result of the reaction of NO with superoxide anion or by S-nitrosylation of regulatory protein groups.

Zorrilla-Zubilete et al., 2010 reviewed the evidences on the role of NO under different physiological and pathological situations and the intracellular mechanisms involved in NO effects (Figure 2).

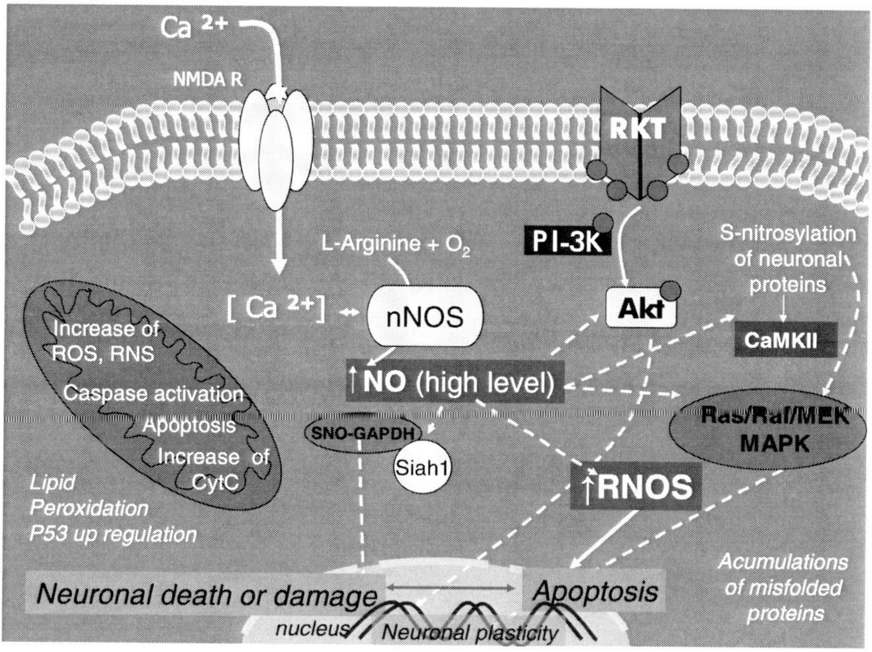

Figure 2. Pathways activated by excessive generation of NO. The s-nitrosylation of GAPDH induces its interaction with Siah 1. When this complex is translocated to the nucleus contributes to neuronal injury and death. The S-nitrosylation of other proteins could exacerbate neuronal injury. High levels of NO may induce apoptosis via caspase family and cytocrome c (Cyt C) activation. Ras/Raf/MEK/ERK pathway, Akt phosphorylation via PI3K and CaMKII can also be stimulated by NO, leading to neuronal damage and/or apoptosis.

Maur et al. showed an increase in calcium-dependent NOS in prenatally stressed animals when compared to control animals. This increase in NO might drive to neurotoxicity mechanisms in the cerebellum, inducing long-term alterations in the circuits involved in memory processes. It is known that a high production of NO induces neurotoxicity by oxidative stress and that it is directly implied in neurodegenerative processes (Maur et al., 2012).

Given the complexity and interactions present in the circuits involved in cognitive processes in the nervous system, the NO system cannot be thought to be the only factor involved in the alterations here described. However, the extense literature reviewed here allow us to suppose that in maternal stress model NO might have an important participation in the alterations in memory and learning processes induced by stress during early development stages, which may be expressed later in life as an altered behavioural outcome..

Neurotrophic Factors

Neurotrophic factors are peptides that promote neuronal development and differentiation, and are expressed in a particular period and region (Korsching 1993). Nerve tissue depends on them for survival and functioning, as neurotrophins are involved in remodeling processes, adaptation and neuronal plasticity. Neurotrophic factors act in autocrine or paracrine manner and can be secreted by neurons that innervate tissues and by glial cells (Korsching 1993). When secreted by the white tissue they act in a retrograde manner favoring the innervation of the afferent neuron. This mechanism involves the secretion of neurotrophic factors into the extracellular space, its capture by a neuron via a specific receptor and internalization of the receptor-peptide complex is transported along the axon to the soma (Korsching 1993).

Neurotrophic factors can also act anterograde being secreted from axons. In fact, some neurotrophic factors can act as neurotransmitters and, conversely, some neurotransmitters can exert a trophic function (Korsching 1993).

A neurotrophic factor may exert different effects on a variety of cell types and can influence neuronal and non-neuronal cells, which involves competition between cells for the factors (Korsching 1993). Different neurotrophic factors have different functions, but may overlap by the convergence of signal transduction pathways (Korsching 1993). However, this redundancy has not been demonstrated, since a neuron may need more than one factor for survival. The best known family of neurotrophic factors is the neurotrophin. This family is composed of Nerve Growth Factor (NGF), Brain-Derived Neurotrophic Factor (BDNF), Neurotrophin 3 (NT3) and the Neurotrophin 4 (NT4) among others.

The first neurotrophin to be characterized in vertebrates was the NGF. Later the BDNF, NT3 and NT4 were discovered. It is a fairly conserved group of proteins that share 50% homology (Binder DK 2004). Neurotrophins are synthesized as pro-hormones which are then cleaved giving rise to the 14 kDa mature form. Finally, two of them combine to form a homo dimer by noncovalent bonds (Blum 2005). NGF, acts in a retrograde manner, while NT3 and BDNF act both retrogade and anterograde (Korsching 1993). All are expressed in the hippocampus (MH Skup. 1994) but BDNF is particularly abundant (Binder DK 2004). There are two types of neurotrophin receptors: the high affinity Trk and low affinity p75. Both membrane receptors establish a cross-talk between each other.

The Trk located in neurons and astrocytes, transmit signals that increase survival and promote cell growth. Troponin-type receptors are receptors with kinase activity (Trk). The receptor p75 belongs to the superfamily of receptors for TNF (tumor necrosis factor) and Fas (focal adhesion kinase), and possesses tyrosine kinase activity. It has similar affinity for all neurotrophins. This receptor promotes neuronal survival, but, under certain conditions, can induce cell death.

Signaling Pathways Activated by Neurotrophins

The Trk receptors are distributed all along the cell body and neurites. Binding of neurotrophins to the receptor induces conformational changes leading to receptor dimerization and activation (Blum 2005). It can trigger signaling cascades from the membrane or may be endocytosed and activate signaling cascades from the vesicle and then being retrogradely transported to the soma. The signaling pathways that can be triggered are (Huang 2001 and Van den Hove, 2012):

- The MAP kinase cascade, which is responsible for a cell survival induced by neurotrophins and is vital for the protection of neurons from oxidative stress and damage by cytokines. This cascade can be activated by growth factors or transcription factors, and may also be involved in the LTP process.
- The phospholipase C (PLCgama) signalling pathway which leads to the depletion of Ca2 + from intracellular reservoirs and the subsequent activation of kinases. This pathway may also be involved in the LTP process.
- Phosphatidylinositol 3'-kinase (PI3K) pathway which is largely responsible for NGF-induced survival. This phenomena is involved in apoptotic cascade, inhibiting procaspase-9 and stimulating the synthesis of pro-apoptotic factor Bcl-2, among others.

The resulting response of neurotrophin-receptor interaction will depend on which route is activated, which may depend on the potency and duration of activation of different receptors and the co-expression of these.

In general, all neurotrophins play a role in the survival, development and differentiation of neurons and neurite growth and influence protein expression essential for normal functioning of neurons. NGF, for example, stimulates survival and neurite initiation (Levi-Montalcini 1963, Katz et al. 1990), and neuritic development (Campenot 1977). It also stimulates the synthesis of various neuropeptides (Kessler JA, 1981, Heumann R 1987) and plays an important role in the maintenance of a differentiated state of neurons and sensory synapsis (Misko TP 1987).

BDNF promotes survival and growth in a variety of neurons. For example, BDNF contributes to the development of activity of the visual cortex (Binder DK 2004), suggesting a role in axonal wiring development. BDNF also has important effects on dendritic morphology (McAllister et al., 1997, Murphy et al., 1998) and promotes neurogenesis (Katoh-Semba et al., 2002).

NT3 has a role in the development and survival of neurons (Huang EJ 2001), development of hippocampal neuronal precursors (Vicar-Abejóon et al. 1995), survival and development of oligodendrocytes (Barres et al. 1994).

Action of the Neurotrophins in the Synapses, Neuronal Plasticity and Behaviour

Both BDNF and NT3 play a role in the synapse. This is a very important function of BDNF, as a promoter of LTP. Hippocampal slices treated with BDNF or NGF and NT3 show a persistent increase in postsynaptic potential amplitude, similar to what happens with the induction of LTP (Kang and Schuman 1995). Conversely, in BDNF knockout mice tetanic stimulation fails to induce LTP, and this is reversed by the addition of exogenous BDNF (Korte et al. 1995; Patterson et al. 1996). Furthermore, electrical stimulations induce LTP and increase expression of BDNF and NGF (Patterson et al., 1992). Some experiments demonstrate that the effect of BDNF on LTP would be at the presinapsis affecting neurotransmitter release, but there is also strong evidence of postsinaptic effects (McKay 1999, Binder DK 2004). In postsinapsis, BDNF modulates the NMDA receptor and GABA channels that activates voltage-dependent sodium channels leading to the release of neurotransmitters from the dendrites (Blum 2005).

It has been demonstrated that induction of the expression of BDNF in hippocampus during contextual learning improves spatial learning (Binder DK 2004, Mizuno M 2000).

Deregulation of neurotrophins is associated with various pathologies of the nervous system. In Alzheimer's and Parkinson's neurodegenerative diseases, BDNF in hippocampus and neocortex (Schindowski K 2008) and in the substantia nigra, respectively (Binder DK 2004) was diminished. In Alzheimer's disease there is an increase of pro-NGF and decrease of TrkA decreased in some areas of the brain. Furthermore, NGF stimulates transcription of the APP peptide (Schindowski K 2008). Hippocampal BDNF expression was increased in epileptic patients (Mathern et al., 1997). In addition, seizures increase levels of NGF messenger (Gall and Isackson, 1989). Treatments with antidepressant drugs and lithium increase BDNF levels (DK Binder 2004). Furthermore, hippocampal BDNF expression increases after brain injury (Lindvall et al. 1992).

A recent review hypothesizes that during gestation, neurotrophins may play numerous roles in angiogenesis, energy homoeostasis, regulation of growth factors actions and development and maturation of the feto-placental unit (Mayeur et al., 2011).

Neurotrophins such as BDNF potentiate the placental development and play an important role in cytotrophoblast differentiation, proliferation and survival (Kawamura et al., 2009, 2011). Abnormal brain development in a compromised prenatal and/or early postnatal environment is thought to be a risk factor for several neurological disorders (Rehn and Rees, 2005). Reports indicate that maternal BDNF reaches the fetal brain through utero-placental barrier and might contribute to its development (Kodomari et al., 2009). BDNF exerts its biological function through binding to its receptor TrkB, which initiates multiple signalling cascades and has been implicated in several neurological disorders like schizophrenia (Hashimoto et al., 2005; Numakawa et al., 2010). (Fig 3). Further, the levels of BDNF are known to be regulated by omega 3 fatty acids (docosahexaenoic acid: DHA) (Wu et al., 2004) (Dhobale et al., 2012). It has been previously shown that prenatal stress in the last week of fetal gestation can produce multiple endophenotypic changes related to schizophrenia in the Sprague–Dawley rat strain (Kinnunen et al., 2003; Koenig et al., 2005; Lee et al., 2007; Taylor et al., 2010). Different rat strains have some differences in their stress response, Fischer rats have a hyperactive HPA-axis, Lewis rats are known to be hypo-responsive to stress, and Sprague–Dawley rats have an intermediate corticosterone response (Dhabhar et al., 1993; Moncek et al., 2001; Kosten and Ambrosio, 2002).

The neurotrophin gene BDNF is associated with several neuropsychiatric disorders, including depression, autism, bipolar disorder, and schizophrenia, and it is an important gene of interest in stress research (Correia et al., 2010; Buckley et al., 2007; Angelucci et al., 2005). BDNF as previously mentioned induces the survival (Hempstead, 2006) development, and function (Reichardt, 2006) of selected neuronal populations of the peripheral and central nervous systems and participate in the modulation of dendritic growth and morphology (Binder and H.E. Scharfman,2004; Bibel and Barde, 2000). In the later stages of nervous system development and in the adult BDNF regulates synaptic transmission and plasticity and acts as a central modulator of pain (Pezet and McMahon, 2006).

BDNF regulates synaptic plasticity in neuronal networks involved in depressive behaviours (Pittenger and Duman, 2007; Schinder and Poo, 2000). Regulation of BDNF may reverse stress-induced deficits in structural and synaptic plasticity in the adult brain, resulting in cognitive flexibility and, subsequently, an increased ability to adapt/cope with environmental challenges that may precipitate or exacerbate depressive episodes (Schmidt, Shelton and Duman, 2011).

BDNF gene has 11 exons and nine functional promoters that are tissue-specific and have activity-dependent regulation across development and in adulthood (Nair et.al, 2007; Aid et.al, 2007; Liu et.al, 2006; Sathanoori et.al, 2004). It is mainly expressed in the central nervous system, particularly in the cortex, hippocampus, and forebrain but it is also found in peripheral tissues (Pruunsild et.al, 2007).

Clinical and experimental studies indicate that the prefrontal cortex (PFC) and hippocampus might play a pivotal role in the cognitive deficits and aberrant emotional behaviours originated from early-life adversity (De Bellis, 2005; Kaffman and Meaney, 2007; Fumagalli et. al, 2007; Noble, Tottenham and Casey, 2005; Teicher et. al, 2003)

Dennis and Levitt (2005) had determined that methylation of exon IV was a likely mechanism mediating BDNF gene expression during development and thus susceptible to environmental insults. Thus, Roth et al. (2009) have evaluated offspring exposed to a stressed-abusive mother (maltreatment) or to a normal maternal care or positive caregiving mother (cross-fostered care). They demonstrate that early experiences of maltreatment increases BDNF DNA methylation at both exons IV and IX within the PFC that persist into adulthood.

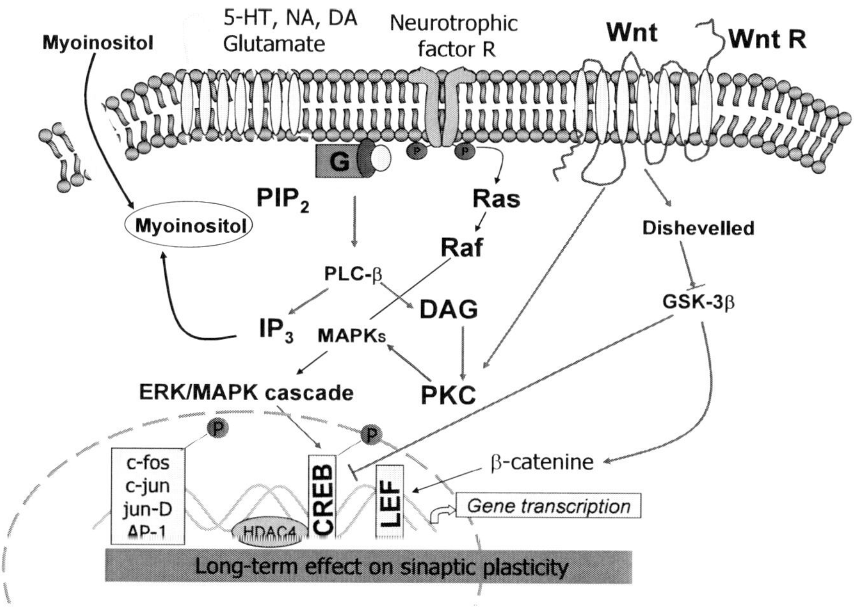

Figure 3. Schematic signaling cascades affected by prenatal stress.

CONCLUSION

The differential effect of prenatal stress on learning and memory ability of males and females probably has a physiological basis that is determined in intrauterine development. Not surprisingly, stress exerted in this period can differentially affect males and females since during intrauterine development there is a brain and neuronal differentiation characteristic of each sex. In fact, the sexual hormones play an important role in the determination of different brain regions, and it is very likely that the intrauterine stress is involved in this process because glucocorticoids play a regulatory effect on the gonads. Furthermore, it should be noted that, particularly, the hippocampus has gonadal hormone receptors. The physiological roles of NO depend on its local concentration as well as availability and the nature of downstream target molecules. NO is a signaling mediator with many diverse and often opposing biological activities. The diversity of responses to this simple molecule comes from the enormous variety of chemical reactions and biological properties associated with it. At low nanomolar concentrations, activation of soluble guanylyl cyclase (sGC) is the major event initiated by NO. Cyclic GMP directly regulates the activities of its downstream effectors such as Protein Kinase G (PKG), Cyclic Nucleotide Gated channels (CNG) and Cyclic nucleotide phosphodiesterases, which in turn regulate the activities of a number of proteins that are involved in modulating diverse cellular and physiological processes. At micromolar concentrations, NO reacts with superoxide anion to form reactive peroxinitrite, thereby leading to the oxidation of important cellular proteins. It has been shown that NO is an important modulator of axon outgrowth and guidance, synaptic plasticity, neuronal precursor proliferation as well as neuron survival. However, excessive nitrosative and oxidative stress, possibly triggered by over activation of NMDA receptors and mitochondrial dysfunction, may affect multiple intracellular signaling pathways that could conceivably contribute to neuronal cell injury and death. It is important to highlight that both positive and negative effects of NO actions have been described. Finally, we conclude that NO and BDNF are important intracellular mediators that can exert both neurotoxic and/or neuroprotective effects in different processes induced by prenatal stress and that it is important to draw a complete picture of its participation in this processes for the development of new therapeutic approaches.

In conclusion, the prenatal stress in different strains of rats or mice is associated with behavioural effects in the offspring. Some studies suggests that resilience to developmental stress exposure may be mediated, at least in part, via nitric oxide and neurotrophins among other intracelullar signalling cascades. Furthermore, these signalling pathways may provide potential targets for novel antidepressant and mood stabilizing drugs treatments, including HDAC inhibitors.

References

Aid T, Kazantseva A, Piirsoo M, Palm K, Timmusk T. Mouse and rat BDNF gene structure and expression revisited. *J Neurosci Res.* 2007, 85:525-535.

Angelucci F, Brene S, Mathe AA. BDNF in schizophrenia, depression and corresponding animal models. *Mol Psychiatry.* 2005; 10:345-352.

Araki T, Tanji H, Fujihara K, et al. 1999. Increases in [3H]FK-506 and [3H]L-NG-nitroarginine binding in the rat brain after nigrostriatal dopaminergic denervation. *Metab Brain Dis;* 14: 21-31.

Barres BA, Raff MC, Gaese F, Bartke I, Dechant G, Barde YA. A crucial role for neurotrophin-3 in oligodendrocyte development. (1994) *Nature*. 367(6461):371-5.

Bibel, Y.A. Barde, Neurotrophins: key regulators of cell fate and cell shape in the vertebrate nervous system, *Genes Dev.* 14 (2000) 2919–2937.

Binder DK, Scharfman HE. Brain-derived neurotrophic factor. (2004) *Growth Factors*. 22(3):123-31.

Blum R, Konnerth A. Neurotrophin-mediated rapid signaling in the central nervous system: mechanisms and functions. (2005) *Physiology* (Bethesda). 20:70-8.

Bobeé S, Mariette E, Tremblay-Leveau H, Caston J. 2000. Effects of early midline cerebellar lesion on cognitive and emotional functions in the rat. *Behavioural Brain Research* 112 (2000) 107–117.

Bowman RE, MacLusky NJ, Sarmiento Y, Frankfurt M, Gordon M, Luine VN. Sexually dimorphic effects of prenatal stress on cognition, hormonal responses, and central neurotransmitters. (2004) *Endocrinology*. 145(8):3778-87.

Bredt DS, Ferris CD, Snyder SH. 1992. Nitric oxide synthase regulatory sites. Phosphorylation by cyclic AMP-dependent protein kinase, protein kinase C, and calcium/calmodulin protein kinase; identification of flavin and calmodulin binding sites. *J Biol Chem*; 267: 10976-81.

Bredt DS, Snyder SH. 1994. Nitric oxide: a physiologic messenger molecule. *Ann Rev Biochem*; 63: 175- 95.

Campenot RB. 1977. Local control of neurite development by nerve growth factor. *Proc Natl Acad Sci U S A*. 1977 Oct;74(10):4516-9.

Caston J, Chianalc C, Delhaye-Bouchaud N, Mariani J. 1998. Role of the cerebellum in exploration behaviour. *Brain Research*. 808:232-237.

Chameau P, Qin Y, Spijker S, Smit G, Joëls M. Glucocorticoids specifically enhance L-type calcium current amplitude and affect calcium channel subunit expression in the mouse hippocampus. (2007) *J Neurophysiol*. 97(1):5-14.

Chen J, Zhang S, Zuo P and Tang L. 1997. Memory-related changes of nitric oxide synthase activity and nitrite level in rat brain. *NeuroReports*. 8:1771-1774.

Correia CT, Coutinho AM, Sequeira AF, Sousa IG, Venda LLO, Almeida JP, Abreu RL, Lobo C, Miguel TS, Conroy J, Cochrane L, Gallagher L, Gill M, Ennis S, Oliveira GG, Vicente AM. Increased BDNF levels and NTRK2 gene association suggest a disruption of BDNF/TrkB signaling in autism. *Genes Brain Behav*. 2010, 9:841-848.

Coyle JT and Puttfarken P. 1993. Oxidative stress, glutamate and neurodegenerative disorders. *Science*. 262: 689-695.

Cui B, Wu M, She X. Effects of chronic noise exposure on spatial learning and memory of rats in relation to neurotransmitters and NMDAR2B alteration in the hippocampus. (2009) *J Occup Health*. 51(2):152-8.

Dawson TM and Snyder SH. 1994. Gases as biological messengers: nitric oxide and carbon monoxide in the brain. *J. Neurosci*. 14: 5147-5159.

Dawson V, Dawson T. 1996. Nitric oxide neurotoxicity. *Journal of Chemical Neuroanatomy*. 10:179-190.

De Bellis MD, The psichobiology of neglect. *Child Maltreat*. 2005; 10:150-172.

de Lima MN, Presti-Torres J, Vedana G, Alcalde LA, Stertz L, Fries GR, Roesler R, Andersen ML, Quevedo J, Kapczinski F, Schröder N. 2011. Early life stress decreases hippocampal BDNF content and exacerbates recognition memory deficits induced by repeated D-amphetamine exposure. *Behav Brain Res*. 224(1):100-6.

Dennis KE, Levitt P. Regional expression of brain derived neurotrophic factor (BDNF) is correlated with dynamic patterns of promoter methylation in the developing mouse forebrain. *Mol Brain Res*. 2005, 140:1-9.

Dhabhar FS, McEwen BS, Spencer RL. 1993. Stress response, adrenal steroid receptor levels and corticosteroid-binding globulin levels--a comparison between Sprague-Dawley, Fischer 344 and Lewis rats. *Brain Res*. 1993 Jul 9;616(1-2):89-98.

Dhobale M, Mehendale S, Pisal, V. D'Souza and S. Joshi. Association of Brain-Derived Neurotrophic Factor and Tyrosine Kinase B Receptor in Pregnancy. *Neuroscience* 216 (2012) 31–37.

Di Monte DA, Royland JE, Anderson A, et al. 1997. Inhibition of monoamine oxidase contributes to the protective effect of 7-nitroindazole against MPTP neurotoxicity. *J Neurochem* 1997; 69: 1771-3.

Dinerman JL, Steiner JP, Dawson TM, et al. 1994. Cyclic nucleotide dependent phosphorylation of neuronal nitric oxide synthase inhibits catalytic activity. *Neuropharmacology* 1994; 33: 1245-51.

Erecinska M, Cherian S, Silver IA. 2004. Energy metabolism in mammalian brain during development. *Prog Neurobiol*. 73(6):397-445. Review.

Fride E, Dan Y, Gavish M, Weinstock M. Prenatal stress impairs maternal behaviour in a conflict situation and reduces hippocampal benzodiazepine receptors. (1985) *Life Sci*. 36(22):2103-9.

Fumagali F, Molteni R, Racagni G, Riva MA. Stress during development: Impact on neuroplasticity and relevance to psychopathology. Prog Neurobiol. 2007; 81:197-217.

Gall CM, Isackson PJ. 1989. Limbic seizures increase neuronal production of messenger RNA for nerve growth factor. *Science.* 1989 Aug 18;245(4919):758-61.

Hashimoto M, Hossain S, Agdul H, Shido O. 2005. Docosahexaenoic acid-induced amelioration on impairment of memory learning in amyloid beta-infused rats relates to the decreases of amyloid beta and cholesterol levels in detergent-insoluble membrane fractions. *Biochim Biophys Acta.* 2005 Dec 30;1738(1-3):91-8. Epub 2005 Dec 28.

Hawkins RD, Son H, Arancio O. 1998. Nitric oxide as a retrograde messenger during long-term potentiation in hippocampus. *Prog Brain Res.*118:155-72. Review.

Heumann R. Regulation of the synthesis of nerve growth factor. (1987) *J Exp Biol.* 132:133-50

Hodgson ZG, Meddle SL, Roberts ML, Buchanan KL, Evans MR, Metzdorf R, Gahr M, Healy SD. 2007. Spatial ability is impaired and hippocampal mineralocorticoid receptor mRNA expression reduced in zebra finches (Taeniopygia guttata) selected for acute high corticosterone response to stress. *Proc Biol Sci.* 22;274(1607):239-45.

Huang EJ, Reichardt LF. Neurotrophins: roles in neuronal development and function. (2001) *Annu Rev. Neurosci.* 24:677-736.

Huang EJ, Reichardt LF. Neurotrophins: roles in neuronal development and function. (2001) *Annu Rev Neurosci.* 24:677-736.

Huttunen MO. Nature. Persistent alteration of turnover of brain noradrenaline in the offspring of rats subjected to stress during pregnancy. (1971) 230(5288):53-5.

Ikeda M, Kawahara S, Kirino Y, Katsuki M, Horie H, Ishikawa Y and Yoshioka T. 2001. Phospholipase Cb4 and Protein Kinase Ca and/or Protein Kinase CbI are involved in the induction of Long Term Depression in cerebellar Purkinje cells. *J Biol Chem* 276, 48: 45236-45242.

Joëls M, Baram TZ. The neuro-symphony of stress. (2009) *Nat Rev Neurosci.* 10(6):459-66.

Kaffman A, Meaney MJ. Neurodevelopmental squelae of postnatal maternal care in rodents. Clinical and research implications of molecular insights. *J Child Psichol Psichiatry.* 2007; 48:224-244.

Kang H, Schuman EM. Long-lasting neurotrophin-induced enhancement of synaptic transmission in the adult hippocampus. (1995) *Science.* 267(5204):1658-62.

Kapoor A, Leen J, Matthews SG. Molecular regulation of the hypothalamic-pituitary-adrenal axis in adult male guinea pigs after prenatal stress at different stages of gestation. (2008) *J Physiol.* 586(Pt 17):4317-26. Epub 2008 Jul 17.

Katoh-Semba R, Asano T, Ueda H, Morishita R, Takeuchi IK, Inaguma Y, Kato K. Riluzole enhances expression of brain-derived neurotrophic factor with consequent proliferation of granule precursor cells in the rat hippocampus. (2002) *FASEB J.* 16(10):1328-30.

Katz DM, Erb M, Lillis R, Neet K. 1990. Trophic regulation of nodose ganglion cell development: evidence for an expanded role of nerve growth factor during embryogenesis in the rat. *Exp Neurol.* 1990 Oct;110(1):1-10.

Kawamura K, Kawamura N, Kumazawa Y, Kumagai J, Fujimoto T, Tanaka T. 2011. Brain-derived neurotrophic factor/tyrosine kinase B signaling regulates human trophoblast growth in an in vivo animal model of ectopic pregnancy. *Endocrinology.* 2011 Mar;152(3):1090-100. doi: 10.1210/en.2010-1124. Epub 2011 Jan 14.

Kawamura K, Kawamura N, Sato W, Fukuda J, Kumagai J, Tanaka T. 2009. Brain-derived neurotrophic factor promotes implantation and subsequent placental development by stimulating trophoblast cell growth and survival. *Endocrinology.* 2009 Aug;150(8):3774-82. doi: 10.1210/en. 2009-0213. Epub 2009 Apr 16.

Kessler JA, Black IB.1981. Nerve growth factor stimulates development of substance P in the embryonic spinal cord. *Brain Res.* 1981 Mar 9;208(1):135-45.

Khaldi A, Chiueh CC, Bullock MR, Woodward JJ. 2002. The significance of nitric oxide production in the brain after injury. *Ann NY Acad Sci;* 962: 53-9.

Kinnunen AK, Koenig JI, Bilbe G. 2003. Repeated variable prenatal stress alters pre- and postsynaptic gene expression in the rat frontal pole. *J Neurochem.* 2003 Aug;86(3):736-48.

Kiss JP, Vizi ES. 2001. Nitric oxide: a novel link between synaptic and nonsynaptic transmission. *Trends Neurosci;* 24: 211-5.

Kodomari I, Wada E, Nakamura S, Wada K. 2009. Maternal supply of BDNF to mouse fetal brain through the placenta. *Neurochem Int.* 2009 Feb;54(2):95-8.

Koenig JI, Elmer GI, Shepard PD, Lee PR, Mayo C, Joy B, Hercher E, Brady DL. 2005. Prenatal exposure to a repeated variable stress paradigm elicits behavioural and neuroendocrinological changes in the adult offspring: potential relevance to schizophrenia. *Behav Brain Res.* 30;156(2):251-61.

Korsching S. The neurotrophic factor concept: a reexamination. (1993) *J Neurosci.* 13(7):2739-48.

Korte M, Carroll P, Wolf E, Brem G, Thoenen H, Bonhoeffer T. Hippocampal long-term potentiation is impaired in mice lacking brain-derived neurotrophic factor. (1995) *Proc Natl Acad Sci U S A.* 1995 Sep 12;92(19):8856-60.

Korte SM, Koolhaas JM, Wingfield JC, McEwen BS. 2005. The Darwinian concept of stress: benefits of allostasis and costs of allostatic load and the trade-offs in health and disease. *Neurosci Biobehav Rev.* 29(1):3-38. Review.

Kosten TA, Ambrosio E. 2002. HPA axis function and drug addictive behaviours: insights from studies with Lewis and Fischer 344 inbred rats. *Psychoneuroendocrinology.* 27(1-2):35-69. Review.

Lee BE, Ha M, Park H, Hong YC, Kim Y, Kim YJ, Ha EH. 2011. Psychosocial work stress during pregnancy and birth weight. *Paediatr Perinat Epidemiol.* 25(3):246-54.

Lee PR, Brady DL, Shapiro RA, Dorsa DM, Koenig JI. 2007. Prenatal stress generates deficits in rat social behaviour: Reversal by oxytocin. *Brain Res.* 2; 1156:152-67.

Lee T, Jarome T, Li SJ, Kim JJ, Helmstetter FJ. Chronic stress selectively reduces hippocampal volume in rats: a longitudinal magnetic resonance imaging study. (2009) *Neuroreport.* 20(17):1554-8.

Lemaire V, Koehl M, Le Moal M, Abrous DN. Prenatal stress produces learning deficits associated with an inhibition of neurogenesis in the hippocampus. (2000) *Proc Natl Acad Sci U S A.* 97(20):11032-7.

Levi-Montalcini R, Angeletti PU. Essential role of the nerve growth factor in the survival and maintenance of dissociated sensory and sympathetic embryonic nerve cells in vitro. (1963) *Dev Biol.* 7:653-9.

Lev-Ram V, Jiang T, Wood J, Lawrence DS, Tsien RY. 1997. Synergies and coincidence requirements between NO, cGMP, and Ca2+ in the induction of cerebellar long-term depression. *Neuron.* 18(6):1025-38.

Li Y, Ji YJ, Jiang H, Liu DX, Zhang Q, Fan SJ, Pan F. Effects of unpredictable chronic stress on behaviour and brain-derived neurotrophic factor expression in CA3 subfield and dentate gyrus of the hippocampus in different aged rats. (2009) *Chin Med J* (Engl). 122(13):1564-9.

Lindvall O, Ernfors P, Bengzon J, Kokaia Z, Smith ML, Siesjö BK, Persson H. 1992. Differential regulation of mRNAs for nerve growth factor, brain-derived neurotrophic factor, and neurotrophin 3 in the adult rat brain following cerebral ischemia and hypoglycemic coma. *Proc Natl Acad Sci U S A*. 15;89(2):648-52.

Lipton SA, Choi Y-B, Pan Z-H, et al. 1993. A redox-based mechanism for the neuroprotective and neurodestructive effects of nitric oxide and related nitroso-compounds. *Nature*; 364: 626-32.

Liu Q-R, Lu L, Zhu X-G, Gong J-P, Shaham Y, Uhl GR. Rodent BDNF genes, novel promoters, novel splice variants and regulation by cocaine. *Brain Res*. 2006, 1067:1-12.

Lonart G, Johanson KM. 1992. Inhibitory effects of nitric oxide on the uptake of [3H]dopamine and [3H] glutamate by striatal synaptosomes. *J Neurochem*; 63: 2108-17.

Maccari S, Darnaudery M, Morley-Fletcher S, Zuena AR, Cinque C, Van Reeth O. Prenatal stress and long-term consequences: implications of glucocorticoid hormones. (2003) *Neurosci Biobehav Rev*. 27(1-2):119-27.

Maccari S, Morley-Fletcher S. Effects of prenatal restraint stress on the hypothalamus-pituitary-adrenal axis and related behavioural and neurobiological alterations. (2007) *Psychoneuroendocrinology*. 32 Suppl 1:S10-5.

Maccari S, Piazza PV, Kabbaj M, Barbazanges A, Simon H, Le Moal M. Adoption reverses the long-term impairment in glucocorticoid feedback induced by prenatal stress. (1995) *J Neurosci*. 15(1 Pt 1):110-6.

Marletta MA. 1994. Nitric oxide synthase: aspects concerning structure and catalysis. *Cell*; 78: 927-30.

Martin L, Goldowitz D, Mittleman G. 2003. The cerebellum and spatial ability: dissection of motor and cognitive components with a mouse model system. *European journal of Neuroscience*. 18:2002-2010.

Martin LA, Escher T, Goldowitz D, Mittleman G. 2004. A relationship between cerebellar Purkinje cells and spatial working memory demonstrated in a lurcher/chimera mouse model system. *Genes Brain Behav*. 3(3):158-66.

Mathern GW, Pretorius JK, Kornblum HI, Mendoza D, Lozada A, Leite JP, Chimelli LM, Fried I, Sakamoto AC, Assirati JA, Lévesque MF, Adelson PD, Peacock WJ. 1997. Human hippocampal AMPA and NMDA mRNA levels in temporal lobe epilepsy patients. *Brain*. 120 (Pt 11):1937-59.

Maur D, Romero C, Palumbo M, Genaro A, Zorrilla Zubilete M. Alterations in behavioural learning due to prenatal stress in rats. (2007) *Biocell*, 31:100.

Maur DG, Romero CB, Burdet B, Palumbo ML, Zorrilla-Zubilete MA. 2012. Prenatal stress induces alterations in cerebellar nitric oxide that are correlated with deficits in spatial memory in rat's offspring. *Neurochem Int.* 2012 Dec;61(8):1294-301.

Mayeur S, Lukaszewski MA, Breton C, Storme L, Junien C, Vieau D, Lesage J. 2011. BDNF in feto-placental development. *Med Sci* (Paris). 27(3):251-2.

McAllister AK, Katz LC, Lo DC. 1997. Opposing roles for endogenous BDNF and NT-3 in regulating cortical dendritic growth. *Neuron.* 18(5):767-78.

McEwen BS. 1998. Stress, adaptation, and disease. Allostasis and allostatic load. *Ann N Y Acad Sci.* 1;840:33-44.

McEwen BS. 1999. Stress and hippocampal plasticity. *Annu Rev Neurosci.;*22:105-22. Review.

McEwen BS. 2007. Physiology and neurobiology of stress and adaptation: central role of the brain. Physiol Rev. 2007 Jul;87(3):873-904. Review.

McKay SE, Purcell AL, Carew TJ. Regulation of synaptic function by neurotrophic factors in vertebrates and invertebrates: implications for development and learning. (1999) *Learn Mem.* 6(3):193-215.

Miranda KM, Espey MG, Wink DA. 2000. A discussion of the chemistry of oxidative and nitrosative stress in cytotoxicity. *J Inorg Biochem*; 79: 237-40.

Misko TP, Radeke MJ, Shooter EM. Nerve growth factor in neuronal development and maintenance. (1987) *J Exp Biol.* 132:177-90.

Mitchell JB, Rowe W, Boksa P, Meaney MJ. Serotonin regulates type II corticosteroid receptor binding in hippocampal cell cultures. (1990) *J Neurosci.* 10(6):1745-52.

Mizuno M, Yamada K, Olariu A, Nawa H, Nabeshima T. 2000. Involvement of brain-derived neurotrophic factor in spatial memory formation and maintenance in a radial arm maze test in rats. *J Neurosci.* 15;20(18):7116-21.

Moncada S, Higgs A. 1993. The L-arginine-nitric oxide pathway. *N Eng J Med*; 329: 2002-12.

Moncada S, Palmer RM, Higgs EA. 1991. Nitric oxide: physiology, pathophysiology and pharmacology. *Pharmacol Rev;* 43: 109-42.

Moncek F, Kvetnansky R, Jezova D. 2001. Differential responses to stress stimuli of Lewis and Fischer rats at the pituitary and adrenocortical level. *Endocr Regul.* 35(1):35-41.

Mueller BR, Bale TL. 2006. Impact of prenatal stress on long term body weight is dependent on timing and maternal sensitivity. *Physiology & Behavior.* 88:605-614.

Muramatsu Y, Kurosaki R, Watanabe H, et al. 2003. Cerebral alterations in a MPTP-mouse model of Parkinson's disease-an immunocytochemical study. *J Neural Transm* 2003; 110: 1129-44.

Murphy DD, Cole NB, Segal M. Brain-derived neurotrophic factor mediates estradiol-induced dendritic spine formation in hippocampal neurons. (1998) *Proc Natl Acad Sci U S A.* 95(19):11412-7.

Nair A, Vadodaria KC, Banerjee SB, Benekareddy M, Dias BG, Duman RS, Vaidya VA. Stressor-specific regulation of distinct brain-derived neurotrophic factor transcripts and cyclic AMP response element-binding protein expression in the postnatal and adult rat hippocampus. *Neurophsychopharmacol.* 2007, 32:1504-1519.

Nakane M, Mitchell J, Forstermann U, Murad F. 1991. Phosphorylation by calcium calmodulin-dependent protein kinase II and protein kinase C modulates the activity of nitric oxide synthase. *Biochem Biophys Res Commun*; 14: 1396- 402.

Nathan C, Xie QW. 1994. Nitric oxide synthases: roles, tolls, and controls. *Cell*; 78: 915-8.

Nathan C, Xie QW. 1994. Nitric oxide synthases: roles, tolls, and controls. *Cell* 1994; 78: 915-8.

Noble KG, Tottenham N, Casey BJ. Neuroscience perspectives on disparities in school readiness and cognitive achievement. *Future Child.* 2005; 15:71-89.

Numakawa T, Kumamaru E, Adachi N, Yagasaki Y, Izumi A, Kunugi H. Glucocorticoid receptor interaction with TrkB promotes BDNF-triggered PLC-gamma signaling for glutamate release via a glutamate transporter. (200) *Proc Natl Acad Sci USA.* 106(2):647-52.

Palumbo ML, Fosser NS, Rios H, Zorrilla Zubilete MA, Guelman LR, Cremaschi GA, Genaro AM. Loss of hippocampal neuronal nitric oxide synthase contributes to the stress-related deficit in learning and memory. (2007) *J Neurochem.* 102(1):261-74.

Passot JB, Sheynikhovich D, Duvelle É, Arleo A. 2012. Contribution of cerebellar sensorimotor adaptation to hippocampal spatial memory. *PLoS One.* 7(4).

Patel PD, Katz M, Karssen AM, Lyons DM. Stress-induced changes in corticosteroid receptor expression in primate hippocampus and prefrontal cortex. (2008) *Psychoneuroendocrinology.* 33(3):360-7.

Patin V, Lordi B, Vincent A, Caston J. 2005. Effects of prenatal stress on anxiety and social interactions in adult rats. *Brain Res Dev Brain Res.* 160(2):265-74.

Patterson SL, Abel T, Deuel TA, Martin KC, Rose JC, Kandel ER. Recombinant BDNF rescues deficits in basal synaptic transmission and hippocampal LTP in BDNF knockout mice. (1996) *Neuron.* 16(6):1137-45.

Patterson SL, Grover LM, Schwartzkroin PA, Bothwell M. Neurotrophin expression in rat hippocampal slices: a stimulus paradigm inducing LTP in CA1 evokes increases in BDNF and NT-3 mRNAs. (1992) *Neuron.* 9(6):1081-8.

Pezet, S.B. McMahon, Neurotrophins: mediators and modulators of pain, *Annu. Rev. Neurosci.* 29 (2006) 507–538.

Pittenger C, Duman RS. Stress, depression, and neuroplasticity: a convergence of mechanisms. *Neuropsychopharmacology*. 2007; 33:88–109.

Pruunsild P, Kazantseva A, Aid T, Palm K, Timmusk T. Dissecting the human BDNF locus: Bidirectional transcription, complex splicing, and multiple promoters, *Genomics*, Volume 90, Issue 3. 2007; 397-406.

Rehn AE, Rees SM. 2005. Investigating the neurodevelopmental hypothesis of schizophrenia. Clin Exp Pharmacol Physiol. 32(9):687-96. Review.

Roth TL, Lubin FD, Funk AJ, Sweat D. Lasting epigenetic influence of early-life adversity on the BDNF Gene. *Biol Pshychiatry*. 2009; 65:760-769.

Ruiz R, Avant C. 2005. Effects of Maternal Prenatal Stress on Infant Outcomes. *Advances in Nursing Science.* 28:345-355 .

Sapolsky RM, Krey LC, McEwen BS. Glucocorticoid-sensitive hippocampal neurons are involved in terminating the adrenocortical stress response. (1984) *Proc Natl Acad Sci U S A.* 81(19):6174-7

Sapolsky RM. Glucocorticoid toxicity in the hippocampus: reversal by supplementation with brain fuels. (1986) *J Neurosci.* 6(8):2240-4.

Sapolsky RM.1992. Do glucocorticoid concentrations rise with age in the rat? *Neurobiol Aging*.13(1):171-4.

Sathanoori M, Dias BG, Nair AR, Banjerjee SB, Tole S, Vaidya VA. Differential regulation of multiple brain-derived neurotrophic factor transcripts in the postnatal and adult rat in hippocampus during development, and in response to kitinate administration. *Brain Res Mol Brain Res.* 2004, 130:170-177.

Schinder AF, Poo M. The neurotrophin hypothesis for synaptic plasticity. Trends Neurosci. 2000; 23:639–645.

Schindowski K, Belarbi K, Buée L. Neurotrophic factors in Alzheimer's disease: role of axonal transport. (2008) *Genes Brain Behav*. 7 Suppl 1:43-56.

Schmidt HD, Shelton RC, Duman RS. Functional biomarkers of depression: diagnosis, treatment, and pathophysiology. *Neuropsychopharmacology*. 2011; 36(12):2375–2394.

Schulz JB, Matthews RT, Muqit MMK. 1995. Inhibition of neuronal nitric oxide synthase by 7- nitroindazole protects against MPTPinduced neurotoxicity in mice. *J Neurochem*; 64: 936-9.

Skup MH. BDNF and NT-3 widen the scope of neurotrophin activity: pharmacological implications. (1994). *Acta Neurobiol Exp* (Wars). 54(2):81-94.

Son GH, Geum D, Chung S, Kim EJ, Jo JH, Kim CM, Lee KH, Kim H, Choi S, Kim HT, Lee CJ, Kim K. Maternal stress produces learning deficits associated with impairment of NMDA receptor-mediated synaptic plasticity. (2006) *J Neurosci*. 26(12):3309-18.

Taylor JP, Hardy J, Fischbeck KH. Toxic proteins in neurodegenerative disease. (2002) *Science*.296(5575):1991-5.

Teicher MH, Andersen SL, Polcari A, Anderson CM, Navalta CP, Kim DM. The neurobiological consequences of earlystress and childhood maltreatment. *Neurosci Biobehav Rev*. 2003; 87:873-904.

Ulupinar E, Yucel F, Ortug G. 2006. The effects of prenatal stress on the Purkinje cell neurogenesis. *Neurotoxicol Teratol*. 28(1):86-94.

Ulupinar E, Yucel F. 2005. Prenatal stress reduces interneuronal connectivity in the rat cerebellar granular layer. *Neurotoxicol Teratol*. 27(3):475-84.

Uno H, Tarara R, Else JG, Suleman MA, Sapolsky RM. 1989. Hippocampal damage associated with prolonged and fatal stress in primates. *J Neurosci*. 9(5):1705-11.

Vallee M, Mayo W, Dellu F, Le Moal M, Simon H and Maccari S. 1997. Prenatal stress induces high anxiety and postnatal handling induces low anxiety in adult offspring: correlation with stress-induced corticosterone secretion. *J Neurosci*. 17:2626–2636.

Van den Hove D, Steinbusch H, Scheepens A, Van de Berg W, Kooiman L, Boosten B, Prickaerts J, Blanco C. 2005. Prenatal stress and neonatal rat brain development. *Developmental Neuroscience*. 27(5):313-20.

Van den Hove D.L.A., Lauder J.M., Scheepens A., Prickaerts J., Blanco C.E., Steinbusch H.W.M. Prenatal stress in the rat alters 5-HT1A receptor binding in the ventral hippocampus (2006) *Brain Res*. 1090(1):29-34.

Van den Hove DL, Kenis G, Brass A, Opstelten R, Rutten BP, Bruschettini M, Blanco CE, Lesch KP, Steinbusch HW, Prickaerts J. 2012. Vulnerability versus resilience to prenatal stress in male and female rats; Implications from gene expression profiles in the hippocampus and frontal cortex. Eur Neuropsychopharmacol. doi:pii: S0924-977X(12)00308-2.

Van Reeth O, Koehl M, Weibel L, Le Moal M, Maccari S. 1998. Effects of prenatal stress on circadian synchronization in adult rats. *J Sleep Res.* 7(Suppl. 2):287.

Vicario-Abejón C, Johe KK, Hazel TG, Collazo D, McKay RD. Functions of basic fibroblast growth factor and neurotrophins in the differentiation of hippocampal neurons. (1995) *Neuron.* 15(1):105-14.

Weinstock M. 2001. Alterations induced by gestational stress in brain morphology and behaviour of the offspring. *Prog Neurobiol.* 65(5):427-51.

Weinstock M. Alterations induced by gestational stress in brain morphology and behaviour of the offspring. (2001) *Prog Neurobiol.* 65(5):427-51.

Wink DA, Vodovotz Y, Grisham MB, et al. 1999. Antioxidant effects of nitric oxide. *Methods Enzymol*; 301: 413-24.

Wu A, Ying Z, Gomez-Pinilla F. 2004. Dietary omega-3 fatty acids normalize BDNF levels, reduce oxidative damage, and counteract learning disability after traumatic brain injury in rats. *J Neurotrauma.* 21(10):1457-67.

Wu J, Song TB, Li YJ, He KS, Ge L, Wang LR. 2007. Prenatal restraint stress impairs learning and memory and hippocampal PKCbetal expression and translocation in offspring rats. *Brain Res.* 13 (1141):205-13.

Wu J, Song TB, Li YJ, He KS, Ge L, Wang LR. Prenatal restraint stress impairs learning and memory and hippocampal PKCbetal expression and translocation in offspring rats. (2007) *Brain Res.* 1141:205-13.

Zhe D, Fang H, Yuxiu S. Expressions of hippocampal mineralocorticoid receptor (MR) and glucocorticoid receptor (GR) in the single-prolonged stress-rats. (2008) *Acta Histochem Cytochem.* 41(4):89-95.

Zheng H, Yang Q, Xu CT. Effects of chronic stress and phenytoin on the long-term potentiation (LTP) in rat hippocampal CA1 region. (2004) *Acta Biochim Biophys Sin* (Shanghai). 36(5):375-8.

Zorrilla-Zubilete MA, Maur DG, Palumbo ML, Genaro AM. 2010. Role of Nitric Oxide Signaling Pathways in Brain Injuries. Current Chemical Biology, 4, 250-261. Bentham Science Publishers Ltd.

Zuena AR, Mairesse J, Casolini P, Cinque C, Alemà GS, Morley-Fletcher S, Chiodi V, Spagnoli LG, Gradini R, Catalani A, Nicoletti F, Maccari S.

2008. Prenatal restraint stress generates two distinct behavioral and neurochemical profiles in male and female rats. *PLoS One*. 3(5):e2170.

In: Neonatal Care: New Research
Editors: F. Koubek and J. Linser
ISBN: 978-1-62618-454-1

Chapter 2

PHOSPHODIESTERASES AND THEIR INHIBITORS IN SOME RESPIRATORY SYSTEM DISORDERS

Juraj Mokry[1]* and Daniela Mokra[2]†
[1]Department of Pharmacology, [2]Department of Physiology,
Jessenius Faculty of Medicine, Comenius University,
Martin, Slovakia

ABSTRACT

Phosphodiesterases (PDEs) represent a super-family of 11 classes of metalophosphohydrolases with ubiquitous occurrence and diverse effect. Their role in different tissues, e.g. smooth muscle, immune cells, as well as in various pathological conditions, e.g. inflammation, cough, airway hyperresponsiveness, pulmonary hypertension suggests a potential use of their inhibitors in respective therapeutic approach. In this chapter, physiological and pathophysiological roles of PDEs are reviewed with possible pharmacological modulation of their activity. Classification and pharmacological characteristics of non-selective and selective PDE inhibitors are described more in detail, e.g. mechanism of action, pharmacokinetics, and adverse effects. Special attention is drawn on use

* Corresponding author: Juraj Mokry, MD, PhD. Department of Pharmacology, Jessenius Faculty of Medicine, Comenius University, Sklabinska 26, 03601 Martin, Slovakia. Phone: +421 43 2633619; E-mail: mokry@jfmed.uniba.sk.
† E-mail: mokra@jfmed.uniba.sk.

of PDE inhibitors in respiratory and inflammatory disorders, like airway hyperresponsiveness and meconium aspiration syndrome, where original experimental results are confronted with published preclinical and clinical data.

Keywords: Phosphodiesterase, theophylline, methylxanthines, selective PDE inhibitors, airways, bronchial asthma, meconium aspiration syndrome

INTRODUCTION

Phosphodiesterases (PDEs) represent a superfamily of enzymes – phosphohydrolases, which are able to catalyze a hydrolysis of 3` cyclic phosphate bonds in cyclic 3`,5` adenosine and/or guanosine monophosphate (cAMP and cGMP).

It is widely known that each type of cells can produce several different PDE subtypes. Thus, their origin and localization are considered as a major regulatory mechanism in concentration of cyclic nucleotides (cAMP and cGMP) in the respective cells and tissues. The main role of PDEs is to control the hydrolysis of cyclic nucleotides. As the regulation of ligand or second messenger degradation leads to more significant and faster changes in its concentration compared to influencing its production, the use of PDE inhibition was very fast appreciated and currently considered as an effective and accepted strategy in the therapy of various diseases. Caffeine was found to be a significant inhibitor of PDE activity. Another member of the group of methylxanthines, theophylline, plays an important role in the therapeutic management of different pulmonary diseases. However, these first non-selective inhibitors have relatively narrow therapeutic index, based not only on their pharmacokinetic properties, but also on their ability to inhibit most of the PDE subtypes in different tissues and organs, i.e. their effect is non-selective regarding the PDE inhibition (Bender and Beavo, 2006).

NON-SELECTIVE PDE INHIBITORS (METHYLXANTHINES)

Xanthine derivatives (methylxanthines) can be found as natural purine alkaloids in several plants, e.g. fruit of coffee and cocoa as well as leaves of tea plant. The most famous methylxanthine, caffeine (1,3,7-trimethylxanthine), was isolated from green coffee bean in Germany in 1820 for the first time.

However, its premiere complete synthesis was successful in 1885 (Nosalova, 2000). Central psychostimulating effects prevail among its effects, contrary to theophylline and theobromine, were peripheral effects (bronchodilating and cardiostimulating) are dominating.

Theophylline has been used in clinical practice for around 80 years. As the most commonly used agent from the group of methylxanthines has relatively narrow therapeutic range. Doses required for reaching plasmatic levels between 5-15 mg/l are considered as safe (Barnes, 2005). However, a significant bronchodilating effect can be observed only in higher plasmatic concentrations (>10 mg/l), whereas anti-inflammatory action can be observed already at the concentration of 5-10 mg/l. Nowadays, theophylline is used predominantly for the therapy of chronic obstructive pulmonary disease (COPD) and bronchial asthma. Nevertheless, a development of newer antiasthma drugs transferred theophylline into a position of additional bronchodilating drug (Barnes, 2005). Except of anti-inflammatory and bronchodilating action, theophylline as well as theobromine have both antitussive activity demonstrated on naïve as well as ovalbumin sensitized guinea pigs (Mokry et al., 2009), and healthy cats (Nosalova and Mokry, 2001).

Aminophylline is a mixture of theophylline and ethylenediamine (ratio 2:1). Thus, the effects of aminophylline are mostly similar to those of theophylline. Ethylenediamine is an additive used for increasing the solubility and thus absorption of theophylline. Furthermore, it has a very efficient antioxidant action, able to scavenge hydroxyls (OH.) and hypochlorous acid (HOCl) in *in vivo* conditions, preventing oxidative burst in tissues (Lapenna et al. 1995). In clinical practice, aminophylline is used for its bronchorelaxing and anti-inflammatory effects, as well as its ability to stimulate breathing (Barnes, 2005, Salari et al., 2005).

Another representative of methyxanthines is pentoxifylline (dimethylxanthine). Pentoxifylline has excellent hemorheologic properties, decreases platelets aggregation, thrombus creation and improves peripheral blood flow. Therefore, it is used in the therapy of *cludicatio intermittens* and dementia of vascular origin. Furthermore, by *in vitro* incubation with meconium, an administration of pentoxifylline led to inhibition of polymorphonuclears and decreased the production of TNFα (Tegtmeyer et al., 2002). In *in vivo* experiments, pentoxifylline administered to piglets with meconium aspiration syndrome (MAS) ameliorated local ventilation/perfusion ratio and prevented an increase of TNFα, proteins and alveolar macrophages in bronchoalveolar lavage fluid. However, it did not influence the accumulation of neutrophils in lungs (Korhonen et al., 2004). Therapy with aminophylline in our experiments significantly ameliorated respiratory parameter compared to non-treated group of rabbits with experimentally induced MAS. Aminophylline led to decreased pulmonary vascular resistance expressed as a percentage of right-to-left pulmonary shunts and central venous pressure, and it increased the oxygenation. Furthermore, aminophylline suppressed pulmonary inflammation and edema, decreased the *in vitro* reactivity of tracheal smooth muscle to histamine and decreased the number of neutrophils in lungs as well as oxidation impairment in lungs compared to non-treated animals with MAS. A significant improvement of these pulmonary functions was observable already 30 minutes after administration of aminophylline (Mokra et al., 2007, Mokra and Mokry, 2010).

Mechanism of Action

An exact mechanism of action of methylxanthines (theophylline will be used as a reference in the following text) is still a subject to discussion. Adding theophylline to human airway smooth muscle strips leads to direct relaxation in *in vitro* conditions and has similar final part of action to β_2-agonists, known as so called functional antagonist, i.e. it prevents and blocks the action of all bronchoconstricting agents (Barnes, 2008a).

It is known that non-selective PDE inhibition leads to an increase in intracellular levels of cAMP and cGMP, leading to broncho- and vasodilation. These effects, however, can be observed only in higher plasmatic concentrations of theophylline. The theophylline induced increase of cAMP can lead to opening the ion maxiK^+ channels, promoting the bronchodilating effect. Besides, theophylline decreases intracellular levels of calcium, acetylcholine and monoamines and decreases release and action of various mediators of inflammation and bronchoconstriction, including prostaglandins. Thanks to structural similarities, theophylline and other representatives of methylxanthines are antagonists of adenosine (purinergic) receptors. Theophylline supports an activity of mast cells and basophils, increases surfactant production and mucocilliar transportation and ameliorates scavenging reactive forms of oxygen (Barnes, 2005, Barnes, 2008a, Barnes 2008b). Similarly to theophylline, pentoxifylline is a nonselective PDE inhibitor (increases cAMP) and antagonist of adenosine receptors; however it can inhibit TNFα and leukotriene synthesis, and to suppress inflammation (Deree et al., 2008, Peters-Golden et al., 2005).

The properties of methylxanthines may differ based on their ability to influence PDE isoenzymes or on the level of their interaction with adenosine recepetors. E.g. pentoxifylline and aminophylline have strong antioxidant activity. Aminophylline reduced neutrophil accumulation in lungs, decreased lipid peroxidation, levels of IL-8 and TNFα, and improved oxygenation in patients during heart valve replacement (Luo et al., 2004)]. Pentoxifylline suppressed oxygen species production via neutrophils after their exposition to TNFα in *in vitro* conditions (Zheng et al., 1990).

Nosalova (2000) summarized and divided the methylxanthines effects into two groups – inhibitory and stimulatory. The table 1 was updated with several new mechanisms and effects (Mokry and Mokra, 2013). Nowadays, different classification is preferred, i.e. based on the reached plasmatic levels or used doses (Barnes, 2005).

Table 1. Inhibitory and stimulatory effects of xanthine derivatives (adapted from Barnes, 2005, Nosalova, 2000, Mokry and Mokra, 2013)

Effects of methylxanthines	
Inhibitory	Stimulatory
↓ PDE activity	↑ activity of mast cells, basophils
↓ Concentration of intracellular Ca^{2+}	↑ mucocilliar transportation
↓ activity of adenosine receptors	↑ phlegm secretion in airways
↓ mediator release	↑ surfactant release
↓ production and effects of prostaglandins	↑ release of interleukin 10
↓ levels of monoamines	↑ scavenging oxygen species
↓ acetylcholine release	↑ epinephrine release
↓ activity of NF-κB (nuclear translocation)	↑ apoptosis
↓ activity of phosphoinositid 3-kinase	↑ activity histone deacetylase

Mechanism of Action at Higher Doses

Despite an existence of several confirmed molecular mechanisms of methylxanthine action, most of them are clinically relevant only at higher plasmatic concentrations (very often > 10 mg/l). There are only few proofs of clinical state amelioration and anti-inflammatory action of methylxanthines at lower concentrations (5-10 mg/l). Major mechanisms exerted in higher concentrations are associated with non-selective PDE inhibition.

Theophylline is relatively weak and non-selective PDE inhibitor. PDEs are responsible for degradation of cyclic nucleotides, leading to increased cytoplasm levels of cAMP and cGMP (Figure 1).

In *in vitro* tests, a relaxing effect of theophylline on airway smooth muscle via PDE3 (as well as PDE4 and 5) inhibition was observed; however, relatively high concentrations of theophylline were required to reach maximal relaxation (Rabe et al., 1995). I an older study, Polson et al. (1978) found only 5-10 % inhibition of PDEs at therapeutic plasmatic concentrations of theophylline. Furthermore, the "non-selectivity" of theophylline action on PDEs is responsible for common unwanted effects, e.g. nausea, vomiting and headache, due to increasing plasmatic levels.

Methylxanthines are known also as potent antagonists of adenosine receptors. Adenosine is a signal nucleoside with mixed physiological function; in airways it can cause bronchoconstriction and chronic inflammation. Adenosine modulates the activity of neutrophils, eosinophils, lymphocytes and macrophages significantly (Spicuzza et al., 2006). As a stimulation of adenosine receptors by ATP leads to bronchoconstriction, their antagonism is considered to be the major mechanism of action of theophylline. Unfortunately, similarly to PDE inhibition, this antagonism of adenosine receptors bears responsibility for serious adverse effects, especially of cardiovascular origin (i.e. heart arrhythmias caused by antagonism of A_1 receptors).

Theophylline possesses also other effects, including increased release of interleukin (IL) 10 known for its anti-inflammatory effects, as its release is typically decreased during inflammation. However, this increase is probably associated with PDE inhibition (Mascali et al., 1996).

Furthermore, theophylline influences transcription via inhibiting the penetration of pro-inflammatory transcription factor – nuclear factor kappa B (NF-κB) into nucleus, thus preventing the expression of "inflammatory genes". As this effect is mediated by PDE inhibition, it can be observed only in higher plasmatic concentrations (Ischiyama et al., 2001).

Other mechanisms manifesting only in higher plasmatic concentrations of theophylline include an inhibition of fosfoinositid-3-kinase (an enzyme responsible for responses to oxidative burst), stimulation of apoptotic process in neutrophils and eosinophils (probably through antagonism of adenosine receptors A_{2A}). An apoptosis of T-lymphocytes can be induced by PDE inhibition (Barnes, 2005). Very high and almost toxic concentrations of theophylline (usually over 20 mg/l) can lead to other effects, like increased levels of circulating catecholamines, inhibition of calcium entry into inflammatory cells, suppression of prostaglandin function and antagonism of tumor necrosis factor alpha (TNFα) (Barnes, 2005).

Mechanism of Action at Lower (Therapeutic) Doses

In therapeutically relevant doses, newer mechanisms of action of methylxanthines can be observed, including histone deacetylase (HDAC) activation (Hansel et al., 2004)]. Glucocorticosteroids are known to suppress expression of inflammatory genes via binding to and thus activating specific glucocorticosteroid receptors. Activated receptors are able to involve HDAC2 into transcription complex of inflammatory genes, leading to its activation and reversal of histone acetylation as well as suppression of genes activated by inflammatory stimuli (Barnes, 2006). Theophylline is increasing the HDAC activity and suppressing the expression of inflammatory genes (Ito et al., 2002). This effect is, however, observed only in lower concentrations of theophylline (around 5 mg/l) and disappears with its increasing. The mechanism of theophylline action on HDAC differs from that of glucocorticosteroids. Latest data suggests HDAC is directly activated, independently from involvement of HDAC2 into transcription complex. A mechanism of this HDAC activation is not yet completely elucidated; however, neither PDE inhibition nor adenosine receptor antagonism is involved (21). Thus, theophylline has potential to unblock the glucocorticosteroids resistance occurring in some patients with bronchial asthma or COPD (Barnes, 2008a).

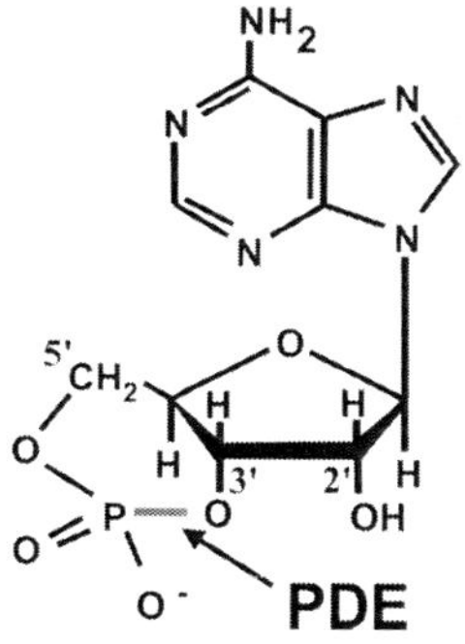

Figure 1. Location of PDE action in cyclic nucleotides.

Adverse Effects

One of the major limitations of wider theophylline use is relatively high occurrence of unwanted effects, especially when crossing its upper therapeutic plasmatic level 15–20 mg/l (Minton and Henry, 1996). Gradational increasing the dose up to a required concentration can prevent them partially. Nevertheless, plasma levels monitoring of theophylline is available and required in most patients.

Interactions at the level of liver metabolism contribute to adverse effects, especially due to theophylline metabolism by a CYP1A2 isoenzyme of P-450 cytochrome. This isoenzyme can be inhibited by macrolides, chinolons, cimetidine, or fluvoxamine, leading to retardation of theophylline metabolism, and thus increasing its plasma levels and occurrence of adverse effects.

The most frequent adverse effects include headache, nausea, vomiting, abdominal pain and restlessness. Increased gastric acid secretion in stomach, gastroesophageal reflux and increased diuresis can be observed, too (Barnes, 2005). Higher concentrations are associated with cramps, changes in cardiovascular parameters (hypertension, tachycardia, increased risk of arrhythmias), and can lead to death (Fakioglu et al., 2004).

Several different mechanisms are involved in adverse effects. Adenosine receptor A_1 antagonism participates in central nervous system stimulation, increased gastric secretion as well as in arrhythmias. Contrary, PDE inhibition (especially PDE4) is involved in development of the most frequent adverse effects, e.g. nausea, gastrointestinal symptomatology, and abdominal pain. These effects can limit the use of the first selective PDE4 inhibitors, as PDE4 influences the vomiting center in brain.

The unwanted effects caused by antagonism of adenosine receptors and PDE inhibition are relatively common at bronchodilating concentrations of theophylline (10-15 mg/l) and they often lead to interruption of the therapy. By using lower concentrations (5-10 mg/l) we can significantly prevent these adverse effects and interactions (Barnes, 2005).

In our experiments in experimentally induced MAS we noticed relatively severe cardiovascular adverse effects associated with intravenous administration of aminophylline. During the first 5 minutes of administration, increased blood pressure and heart rate was observed, followed by increase of several heart rate variability parameters characterizing a parasympathetic activity (Mokra et al., 2013).

There are available several ways, how to prevent adverse effects of aminophylline, or theophylline. 1) The first one is to decrease the drug dosing.

We compared a therapeutic effect of high dose (2 mg/kg) and low dose (1 mg/kg) of aminophylline on pulmonary functions – the results showed more pronounced improvement of some respiratory parameters in high doses; contrary, a decrease of several markers of oxidative stress as well as *in vitro* reactivity of pulmonary strips to bronchoconstricting mediators were more significant in the group of rabbits with lower aminophylline dose (Mokra et al., 2008b). 2) Another way how to prevent adverse effect of aminophylline is to use it in a combination with suitable drugs, e.g. with glucocorticosteroid. An additive effect of both agents enables administration of lower doses and thus decreasing their adverse effects. In our experiments we demonstrated a superior effectiveness of a combination of aminophylline and intratracheally administered budesonide compared to aminophylline alone (Mokra et al. 2008a). 3) Recent therapeutic approaches introduced in order to prevent cardiovascular adverse effects include an administration of selective PDE inhibitors; targeted selectivity to specific PDE isoforms should lead to minimization of adverse effects induced by nonselective PDE inhibition as well as by previously mention mechanisms of methylxanthines independent on PDE inhibition.

Selective PDE Inhibitors

In mammals, there are several PDE subtypes/isoforms, each of them having own structure of active site. Many of PDE isoforms are associated with different body functions as well as with various pathological conditions. Thus it is suggested, selective PDE inhibitors are able to influence different functions and pathological conditions without affecting other organs, or systems and without occurrence of considerable non-specific adverse effects.

Nowadays, PDEs are classified into 11 super families, assembling 21 gene products. Nevertheless, there is an estimation of existing more than 100 different mRNA products (Bender and Beavo, 2006). As the localization of the PDE isoforms is so specific, the function of respective enzyme depends on function of original tissue or organ. Therefore, their selective inhibition can lead to more focused influence on respective tissue/organ in physiological, and especially in pathological condition. Table 2 summarizes currently known functions of PDE isoforms.

While methylxanthines are characteristic for their non-selective PDE inhibition, there are several selective PDE inhibitors with successful experimental and clinical "experience". The mostly studied selective PDE inhibitors related to immune responses in respiratory system are isoforms PDE 3, 4, 5, and 7.

PDE3 Inhibitors

PDE3 is an enzyme hydrolyzing specifically cAMP and occurring in two major isoforms – PDE3A, and PDE3B (Shakur et al., 2001). Nowadays, PDE3 inhibitors are clinically used as non-glycoside cardiotonic drugs – their effect is directly related to selective PDE3A inhibition, known as a cardiovascular type. The major representatives are e.g. amrinon, milrinon, and vesnarinon.

PDE3 activity in respiratory system is exerted predominantly in alveolar macrophagues, endothelial cells, platelets and airway smooth muscle cells. PDE3, together with PDE4, are considered as the most important isoforms hydrolyzing cAMP in airways (Chung, 2006). Except of direct relaxing effect, which is more pronounced after administration of selective PDE3 inhibitors compared to PDE4 inhibitors, PDE3 inhibition leads to enhancement of relaxation evoked by stimulation of β_2-receptors. Furthermore, simultaneous administration of siguazodan (PDE3 inhibitor) and rolipram (PDE4 inhibitor) led to enhancement of this relaxation, suggesting a synergism and possible benefit of parallel PDE3 and PDE4 inhibition. Contrary, PDE3 inhibitors have only weak effect on T-cells activation (Giembycz et al., 1996); however, they can enforce this kind of effect typical for PDE4 inhibitors.

In experimental conditions an antitussive effect of PDE3 inhibitor (cilostazol) was confirmed (Mokry et al., 2008), especially in ovalbumin-sensitized animals. Furthermore, another study by Koike et al. (2008) showed anti-inflammatory action of olprinon (a PDE3 inhibitor) in experimentally induced acute lung injury. Based on these data, PDE3 inhibitors were suggested to be used in some neonatal diseases, like MAS. Milrinone (PDE3 inhibitor) improved oxygenation index and survival rate in 4 patients with MAS (Bassler et al., 2006).

Another PDE3 inhibitor (olprinone) ameliorated pulmonary functions in rabbits with MAS, prevented pulmonary edema, decreased neutrophil count in lungs and the percentage of right-to-left shunts [own unpublished observation]. Further analysis of oxidative stress markers in lungs mitochondria showed significant decrease of lipid and protein oxidation both in lung homogenate and in isolated mitochondria in the olprinone treated group of rabbits with MAS (Mokra et al., 2012). These observations suggest possible benefit of selective PDE inhibitors; however, further analyses are necessary, including other PDE inhibitors (e.g. PDE4).

Table 2. Functions of PDE isoforms (adapted from Bender and Beavo, 2006 and Mokry and Mokra, 2013). Abbreviations: PKA – protein kinase A, NO – nitric oxide

PDE family	Function
PDE1	PDE1A – regulation of vascular smooth muscle, sperm function PDE1B – involved in dopaminergic transmission, influence on surviving and activation of immune cells PDE1C – essential for proliferation of vascular smooth muscle, regulates sperm and neuronal functions
PDE2	PDE2 – mediates connection between cGMP and cAMP metabolism, regulates secretion of aldosterone from suprarenal glad, phosphorylation of Ca^{2+} channels in heart via cAMP and PKA, and via cGMP in neurons, long-term memory, barrier function of endothelial cells in inflammation
PDE3	PDE3A – regulates myocardium contractility, platelets aggregation, vascular and airway smooth muscle contraction, maturation of oocyte and rennin release PDE3B – mediates response to insulin (especially its antilipolytic action), regulates cell cycle/proliferation and mediates inhibitory effects of leptin and other influences on insulin and rennin secretion
PDE4	PDE4 – plays an important role in wide spectrum of processes, almost in all tissues, including neural functions, activation of monocytes and macrophages, infiltration of neutrophils, proliferation of vascular smooth muscle cells, fertility, vasodilation and myocardium contractility
PDE5	PDE5 – regulates vascular smooth muscle in penis and lungs, is involved in mediation of NO-cGMP in platelets (clotting control) and plays role in regulation of cGMP mediation in brain
PDE6	PDE6 – is involved in signal transmission and photoreaction in eye, regulates melatonin release from epiphysis
PDE7	PDE7 – plays a probable role in activation of T-cells as well as other inflammatory cells
PDE8	PDE8 – plays a role in activation of T-cells as well as in function of sperm and Leydig`s cells
PDE9	PDE9 – its role is not completely elucidated, influences signal pathway NO-cGMP in brain
PDE10	PDE10A – regulates cGMP in brain and can play a role in learning and memory processes
PDE11	PDE11 – plays a potential role in development of sperm function

PDE4 Inhibitors

PDE4 enzyme family is encoded in 4 different genes (PDE4A, PDE4B, PDE4C, PDE4D). Products of all four genes specifically hydrolyze cAMP. Except of PDE4C, all of them are expressed in inflammatory cell, e.g. T-cells, B-cells, eosinophils, neutrophils, airway epithelial cells and endothelial cells (Houslay and Adams, 2003). Therefore, the action of selective PDE4 inhibitors is predominantly anti-inflammatory and immunomodulating (Sanz et al., 2005).

One of representatives of the first generation is rolipram. It is a highly selective PDE4 inhibitor, widely used in experimental medicine, inhibiting neutrophil and eosinophil inflammation, interleukin secretion from activated T-helper cells (Th-1 and Th-2), airway epithelial cells, basophils, monocytes and macrophages (Sanz et al., 2005). Despite the inhibition of PDE4 leads to suppression of neutrophil, eosinophil, monocytes and basophil functions, the maximal decrease of macrophage activity and relaxation of airway smooth muscle can be reached only with so called dual effects, i.e. via simultaneous PDE3 and PDE4 inhibition.

Unfortunately, rolipram causes nausea and vomiting relatively frequently, leading to disqualifying it from clinical use. That why newer selective PDE4 inhibitors were tested. As was previously described (Chung, 2006)], nausea and vomiting is a result of activating the high-affinity binding site of PDE for rolipram, whereas anti-inflammatory properties are associated with binding to low-affinity binding site. Newer agents have similar affinity to both of these binding sites, ensuring stronger bronchodilating and anti-inflammatory activity with lower incidence of adverse effects (Chung, 2006). As a representative of this newer – second generation of PDE4 inhibitors, introduced for decreasing the adverse effects, roflumilast, cilomilast and piclamilast should be mentioned. Except of previously mentioned general effects of selective PDE4 inhibitors, these agents are able to decrease the airway hyperreactivity, release of TNF-α, fibrotization and remodeling the pulmonary parenchyma. The reason for that is probably an inhibition of special matrix metalloproteinases as well as other mechanisms, especially in chronic inflammation associated with bronchial asthma and COPD (Chung, 2006). Based on positive results in phase III of clinical drug testing, they were recently introduced into clinical practice for treatment of moderate to severe COPD (Rabe et al., 2005, Matera et al., 2011)

Despite homological natural affinity between special PDE4 subtypes, current trend is to look for even more selective PDE4 inhibitors, potentially active only in special PDE4 subtype. Nevertheless, even already known PDE4 inhibitors have different affinity to respective PDE4 subtypes, leading to diverse occurrence of adverse effects. In our experiments we confirmed potential of PDE4 inhibitors in allergic inflammation; both rolipram and citalopram, representatives of first generation of PDE4 inhibitors, showed suppressive effect on *in vivo* and *in vitro* airway reactivity to histamine in ovalbumin-sensitized guinea pigs (Mokry et al., 2008).

It is necessary to notice that bronchodilating and anti-inflammatory effects of PDE4 inhibitors can be amplified by simultaneous administration of PDE3 inhibitors, suggesting potential benefit of agents with dual action, i.e. inhibiting both PDE3 and PDE4 isoforms.

PDE5 Inhibitors

Contrary to PDE3 and PDE4 inhibitors, PDE5 inhibitors are inactivating cGMP. PDE5 and PDE1 are considered as the major degrading enzymes of cGMP in vascular smooth muscle. PDE5 is expressed in smooth muscle of vascular vessels (especially pulmonary arteries and veins as well as bronchial vessels) and in airway smooth muscle (Sebkhi et al., 2003).

Thus, PDE5 inhibition leads to reduction of pulmonary vascular resistance (Karatza et al., 2005, Sastry et al., 2004), decrease of pulmonary hypertension, and suppression of vascular remodeling (Sebkhi et al., 2003). These effects were observed after stimulation of cGMP production as well as by PDE5 inhibition with sildenafil, leading also to inhibition of cell proliferation and supporting apoptosis (Wharton et al., 2005)]. Therefore, use of PDE5 inhibitors in COPD is tested. Except of previously mentioned, PDE5 inhibitors were shown to have anti-inflammatory effects similar to PDE4 inhibitors (Toward et al., 2004).

In our experiments we showed antitussive effect of zaprinast (PDE5 inhibitor), which was more significant in ovalbumin-sensitized guinea pigs. However, this effect was accompanied only with mild bronchodilating action *in vivo* and non-significant suppression of *in vitro* airway reactivity, suggesting an involvement of other mechanisms in its antitussive effect apart from relaxation of smooth muscle (probably anti-inflammatory action or direct modulation of cough receptors in airways) (Mokry and Nosalova, 2011). Nevertheless, this finding is in concordance with results of Sebkhi et al.(2003), who did not show any effect of zaprinast on bronchodilation and eosinophil accumulation. Conversely, sildenafil as a newer PDE5 inhibitor, led to a significant inhibition of bronchial hyperresponsiveness, leukocyte infiltration and levels of exhaled NO (Toward et al., 2004). This suggests a possible usefulness of PDE4/5 combination in bronchial asthma and COPD therapy.

There were only few selective PDE inhibitors tested in experimentally induced MAS. Except of previously mentioned olprinone (PDE3 inhibitor), PDE5 seems to be a promising target. An administration of sildenafil (PDE5 inhibitor) reversed a blood pressure increase in *arteria pulmonalis* within 1 hour after its administration in piglets with MAS. Furthermore, there was no observable influence on systemic circulation in these animals (Shekerdemian et al., 2002).

PDE7 Inhibitors

PDE7 enzymes are cAMP specific but insensitive to rolipram. Its expression was demonstrated in T-cells, brain as well as skeletal muscle cells (Castro et al., 2005, Smith et al., 2003). PDE7 enzymes are encoded by two genes PDE7A and PDE7B with significant expression of PDE7A1 protein in T-cell lines, peripheral T-lymphocytes, epithelial cell lines, airway and vascular smooth muscle cells, lung fibroblasts, and eosinophils (Ghosh et al., 2009). Thus, the inhibition of this isoenzyme could be an effective tool in suppressing the airway hyperresponsiveness and inflammation. There are several selective PDE7 inhibitors, like e.g. VP1.15 and S14 synthesized in the Instituto de Quimica Medica (Paterniti et al., 2011), pyrimidine inhibitors (Guo et al., 2009), purine inhibitors (Pitts et al., 2004), ASB16165 synthesized in Asubio Pharma Co Ltd in Japan (Kadoshima-Yamaoka et al., 2009), thiadiazol derivative PF0332040 synthesized by Pfizer (Jones et al., 2007). Another selective PDE4 inhibitor has some activity against PDE7 isoenzyme – T-2585 synthesized by the Discovery Research Laboratory in Japan (Nakata et al., 2002). BRL50481 is the only commercially available selective PDE7 inhibitor (Smith et al., 2004). It was previously found to be effective in suppression of some inflammatory cells in *in vitro* conditions, like human monocytes, lung macrophages, and CD8+ T-lymphocytes (Smith et al., 2004). Furthermore, some other roles were recently found, i.e. protection of dopaminergic neurons in animal models of Parkinson disease (Morales-Garcia et al., 2011). In our experiments intraperitoneal administration of BRL50481 led to significant decrease of *in vivo* airway reactivity as well as in *in vitro* conditions. The most significant drop of contractile responses to histamine was observed in ovalbumin-sensitized animals (Christensen et al., 2012). This suggests its potential use in clinical states associated with allergic inflammation, which was mimicked by ovalbumin sensitization. However, an anti-inflammatory action of selective PDE7 inhibitor BRL 50481 administered in monotherapy is relatively weak. Contrary, the combination of PDE7 and PDE4 inhibitor (e.g. BRL 50481 and rolipram) in half doses potentiated the effect observed by single administration of PDE4 as well as PDE7 inhibitors in double doses (based on own unpublished data as well as data published by other authors, (Fortin et al., 2009)). This observation is very important regarding a possible decrease of PDE4 inhibitor dose and thus preventing possible adverse effects (Barnes, 2008a). This concept was described in literature and new dual PDE inhibitors are studied (e.g. PDE3/4 and PDE4/7) for their anti-inflammatory action (Giembycz, 2005b).

Dual and Multi-isoform PDE Inhibitors

A list of available selective PDE inhibitors as well as their potential use can be found in table 3.

Except of selective PDE inhibitors described above, there are numerous multi-isoform inhibitors, i.e. their selectivity is "imperfect" and they are able to inhibit several PDE isoforms (Giembycz, 2005a). Thus, a suitable combination of inhibiting more isoforms (e.g. PDE3 and 4, or PDE4 and 7) could positively potentiate their action in some pathological conditions and minimize their adverse effects through decreased doses (Bender and Beavo, 2006, Giembycz, 2005b). Zardaverine (inhibiting PDE3 and 4), YM-393059 (inhibiting PDE4 and 7), dipyridamol (inhibiting PDE5, 6, 7, 8, 10 and 11) or trequinsin (inhibiting PDE4 and 3) belong to this group of agents. An administration of a drug with dual inhibitory effect on PDE4 and PDE7, e.g. YM-393059, can be considered as a very promising therapeutic tool (Yamamoto et al., 2006). These agents are able to inhibit T-cells functions, i.e. they decrease production and release of cytokines, proliferation and activation of various inflammatory mediators. Stepwise development and tests of dual PDE4-PDE7 inhibitors led to classification of a new independent group of PDE inhibitors, where especially blocking the T-cells functions due to PDE7 inhibition and anti-inflammatory effect due to PDE4 inhibition are expected. Furthermore, these drugs have lower risk of adverse effects (like nausea and vomiting) compared to selective PDE4 inhibitors administered alone, especially due to decreased doses required to reach the same effect.

Contrary, multi-isoform inhibition can result in various adverse effects, which would not be present with "pure" selectivity. Sildenafil (inhibiting PDE1, 5 and 6), tadalafil (inhibiting PDE5, 6 and 11) or vardenafil (inhibiting PDE5 and 6) serve as an example.

CURRENT CLINICAL USES OF PDE INHIBITORS

There are several groups of drugs used in the therapy of obstructive inflammatory airway diseases. They are generally classified as relievers and controllers. Short-acting β_2-agonists and muscarinic antagonists (anticholinergics) belong to the group of relievers, whereas the major controllers, suppressing inflammation, represent glucocorticosteroids, as well as long-acting β_2-agonists and non-selective PDE inhibitors (methylxanthines, e.g. theophylline) with sustained release. Inhalation routes of administration are preferred (except of methylxanthines), associated with significantly reduced incidence of adverse effects. Despite of that, the adverse effects together with limited action in case of lower (safer) doses lead to further development and seeking new drugs suitable for treatment of COPD and bronchial asthma.

In COPD, the major focus is on selective PDE4 inhibitors. Several representatives of 2nd generation are already in clinical phase of drug testing (roflumilast, cilomilast, piclamilast), with roflumilast being registered for severe COPD as an add-on therapy with glucocorticosteroids in 2010 (European Medicines Agency, 2010). Their effectiveness after peroral administration is similar with theophylline, but with relatively lower incidence of adverse effects (Rennard et al., 2008). These are predominantly in gastrointestinal tract (e.g. nausea, diarrhea, as well as headache) and, contrary to theophylline, they do not require therapeutic drug monitoring. Nevertheless, occurrence of these side effects limits increasing their doses (as well as anti-inflammatory potential). An inhalation administration reduced adverse effects; however, it was associated with a decrease of their effectiveness under required level (Barnes, 2008b). Post-marketing surveillance will demonstrate in larger clinical use, whether PDE4 inhibitors will be used only in combination with other anti-inflammatory agents (glucocorticosteroids), or also as monotherapy (Currie et al., 2008). Some carefulness should be kept in mind, as there were recently published negative results of a study with new inhalatory PDE4 inhibitor UK-500,001 (Vestbo et al., 2009). Contrary, studies with oglemilast and Zl-n-91 brought positive results in experimental phase of testing (Spina, 2008, Wang et al., 2010).

Table 3. List of available PDE inhibitors and their major clinical use (updated from Bender and Beavo, 2006, Mokry and Mokra, 2013)

PDE	Inhibitor	Use (actual or under testing)
PDE1	Vinpocetin IC224	Amelioration of blood flow in central nervous system (CNS), amelioration of cognitive functions
PDE2	EHNA BAY 60-7550	Amelioration of memory, decreased endothelium permeability in inflammation
PDE3	Cilostamid Milrinon Cilostazol Olprinon	Therapy of acute heart failure, therapy of *claudicatio intermittens*
PDE4	Rolipram Citalopram Roflumilast Cilomilast Piclamilast Ro 20-1724	Therapy of COPD and other diseases associated with inflammation, impairment of CNS, depression, amelioration of memory
PDE5	Zaprinast Sildenafil Vardenafil Tadalafil	Therapy of erectile dysfunction, therapy of pulmonary hypertension, therapy of acute lung injury, therapy of benign prostatic hyperplasia
PDE6		Possible source of sildenafil adverse effects on vision, not tested as therapeutic target yet
PDE7	BRL 50481 IC242	Anti-inflammatory effects (*in vitro*), *in vivo* use limited so far
PDE8		Completely selective inhibitors not yet available
PDE9	BAY 73-6691	Preclinical tests in the therapy of Alzheimer`s disease
PDE10		Completely selective inhibitors not yet available
PDE11		Inhibited by tadalafil, possible source of adverse effects

Selective PDE4 inhibitors are tested also in bronchial asthma (Hanania, 2008). There are the first clinical trials with roflumilast and cilomilast in athma patients (Hogate, 2009). The experience in children is limited to the theophylline; however, its administration is recommended only in a failure of therapy with first line anti-inflammatory drugs.

Generally, in most developed countries, theophylline is considered as the third line therapy used only in severe bronchial asthma and COPD. Its advantage is a peroral administration and a relatively low price, as well as strong anti-inflammatory action observable in lower, less toxic doses (Diamant et al., 2007) (see above). In children was demonstrated a benefit of aminophylline (theophylline with ethylenediamine) compared to salbutamol in young asthmatics: after an intravenous administration in severe asthma, similar effectiveness was observed with shorter stay in hospital in theophylline group of patients (Roberts et al., 2003). Despite this observation, the last edition of GINA (guidelines for bronchial asthma therapy) characterized effects of regularly administered theophylline as weak and non-significant, nevertheless with amelioration of clinical condition of patients (Global strategy, 2011). As the effectiveness of theophylline is lower compared to low doses of inhalatory glucocorticosteroids, the concomitant occurrence of adverse effects led to classification into D category according to evidence-based medicine.

The use of PDE inhibitors in meconium aspiration syndrome or in acute lung injury in newborns is mostly at experimental level (DeVisser et al., 2008, Mokra and Mokry, 2007, Mokra and Mokry, 2010).

CONCLUSION

Development of selective PDE inhibitors is sometimes characterized only as increasing the selectivity of theophylline, which is already for decades used in clinical practice as a bronchodilator for the therapy of bronchial asthma and COPD. However, theophylline has only weak and non-selective inhibitory action on PDEs, with much more mechanisms of action conditioning its clinical effects. Therefore, selective PDE4 inhibitors can never be categorized as successors of theophylline. Their broad clinical application requires further particular clinical testing, to confirm not only higher effectiveness, but also reduced incidence of adverse effects compared to non-selective PDE inhibitors. Nevertheless, this pharmacological group showed great potential in influencing several respiratory system diseases, especially those associated with chronic inflammation.

ACKNOWLEDGMENTS

Supported by projects "Center of Experimental and Clinical Respirology (CEKR1 and CEKR2), co-financed from EU sources, and by grants of Ministry of Education in Slovak Republic VEGA 1/0030/11 and 1/0057/11.

REFERENCES

Barnes, P.J. (2005). Theophylline in chronic obstructive pulmonary disease. New horizons. *Proc Am Thorac Soc*, 2, 334-9.

Barnes, P.J. (2006). Reduced histone deacetylase in COPD: clinical implications. *Chest*, 129, 151-5.

Barnes, P.J. (2008). Frontrunners in novel pharmacotherapy of COPD. *Curr Opinion Pharmacol*, 8, 300-7.

Barnes, P.J. (2008). Future treatments for chronic obstructive pulmonary disease and its comorbities. *Proc Am Thorac Soc*, 5, 857-64.

Bassler, D., Choong, K., McNamara, P., Kirpalani, H. (2006). Neonatal persistent pulmonary hypertension treated with milrinone: four case report. *Biol Neonate*, 89, 1-5.

Bender, A.T., Beavo, J.A. (2006). Cyclic nucleotide phosphodiesterases: Molecular regulation to clinical use. *Pharmacol Rev*, 58, 488-520.

Castro, A., Jerez, M.J., Gil, C., Martinez, A. (2005). Cyclic nucleotide phosphodiesterases and their role in immunomodulatory responses: advances in the development of specific phosphodiesterase inhibitors. *Med Res Rev*, 25, 229-44.

Christensen, I., Miskovicova, H., Porvaznik, I., Joskova, M., Mokra, D., Mokry, J. (2012). Selective inhibition of phosphodiesterase 7 (PDE7) by BRL50481 in healthy and ovalbumin-sensitized guinea pigs. *Acta Med Martiniana*, 12, 16-23.

Chung, K.F. (2006). Phosphodiesterase inhibitors in airways disease. *Eur J Pharmacol*, 533, 110-7.

Currie, G.P., Butler, C.A., Anderson, W.J., Skinner, C. (2008). Phosphodiesterase 4 inhibitors in chronic obstructive pulmonary disease: a new approach to oral treatment. *Br J Clin Pharmacol*, 65, 803-10.

De Visser, Y.P., Walther, F.J., Laghmani, E.H., Van Wijngaarden, S., Nieuwland, K., Wagenaar, G.T.M. (2008). Phosphodiesterase-4 inhibition attenuates pulmonary inflammation in neonatal lung injury. *Eur Respir J*, 31, 633-44.

Deree, J., Martins, J.O., Melbostad, H., Loomis, W.H., Coimbra, R. (2008). Insights into the Regulation of TNF-α Production in Human Mononuclear Cells: The Effects of Non-Specific Phosphodiesterase Inhibition. *Clinics (Sao Paulo)*, 63, 321–8.

Diamant, Z., Boot, J.D., Virchow, J.C. (2007). Summing up 100 years of asthma. *Respir Med*, 101, 378-88.

European Medicines Agency. European Public Assessment Report (EPAR) for Daxas. [online] 2010 [cited 2012 11 24]. Available from: http://www.ema.europa.eu/ema/index.jsp?curl=pages/medicines/human/medicines/001179/human_med_001363.jsp.

Fakioglu, H., Gelvez, J., Torbati, D., Glover, M.L., Olarte, J.L., Camacho, M.T., Wolfsdorf, J. (2004). Aminophylline therapy during endotoxemia in anesthetized spontaneously breathing rats. *Pharm Res*, 49, 45-50.

Fortin, M., D`Anjou, H., Higgins, M.E., Gougeon, J., Aube, P., Moktefi, K., Mouissi, S., Seguin, S., Seguin, R., Renzi, P.M., Paquet, L., Ferrari, N. (2009). A multi-target antisense approach against PDE4 and PDE7 reduces smoke-induced lung inflammation in mice. *Respiratory Res*, 10, 39.

Ghosh, R., Sawant, O., Ganpathy, P., Pitre, S., Kadam, V.J. (2009). Phosphodiesterase inhibitors: their role and implications. *Int J PharmTech Res*, 1, 1148-60.

Giembycz, M.A. (2005a). Phosphodiesterase-4: Selective and Dual-Specificity Inhibitors for the Therapy of Chronic Obstructive Pulmonary Disease. *Proc American Thor Soc*, 2, 326-33.

Giembycz, M.A. (2005b). Life after PDE4: overcoming adverse events with dual-specificity phosphodiesterase inhibitors. *Curr Opin Pharmacol*, 5, 238-44.

Giembycz, M.A., Corrigan, C.J., Seybold, J., Newton, R., Barnes, P.J. (1996). Identification of cyclic AMP phosphodiesterases 3, 4 and 7 in human $CD4^+$ and $CD8^+$ T-lymphocytes: role in regulating proliferation and the biosynthesis of interleukin-2. *Br J Pharmacol*, 118, 1945-58.

Global strategy for the diagnosis and management of asthma in children 5 years and younger [online]. 2011 [cited 2012 11 24]. Available from: http://www.ginasthma.org

Guo, J., Watson, A., Kempson, J., Carlsen, M., Barbosa, J., Stebbins, K., Lee, D., Dodd, J., Nadler, S.G., McKinnon, M., Barrish, J., Pitts, W.J. (2009). Identification of potent pyrimidine inhibitors of phosphodiesterase 7

(PDE7) and their ability to inhibit T cell proliferation. *Bioorganic Medicinal Chemistry Letters*, 19, 1935-8.

Hanania, N.A. (2008). Targeting airway inflammation in asthma – current and future therapies. *Chest*, 133, 989-98.

Hansel, T.T., Tennant, R.C., Tan, A.J., Higgins, L.A., Neighbour, H., Erin, E.M., Barnes, P.J. (2004). Theophylline: mechanism of action and use in asthma and chronic obstructive pulmonary disease. *Drugs Today*, 40, 55-69.

Holgate, S.T. (2009). Novel targets of therapy in asthma. *Curr Opinion Pulmonary Med*, 15, 63-71.

Houslay, M.D., Adams, D.R. (2003). PDE4 cAMP phosphodiesterase: modular enzymes that orchestrate signalling cross-talk, desensitization and compartmentalization. *Biochem J*, 370, 1-18.

Ischiyama, T., Hasegawa, S., Matsubara, T., Hayashi, T., Furukawa, S. (2001). Theophylline inhibits NF-κB activation and IκBα degradation in human pulmonary epithelial cells. *Naunyn Schmiedebergs Arch Pharmacol*, 364, 558-61.

Ito, K., Lim, S., Caramori, G., Cosio, B., Chung, K.F., Adcock, I.M., Barnes, P.J. (2002). A molecular mechanism of action of theophylline: induction of histone deacetylase activity to decrease inflammatory gene expression. *Proc Natl Acad Sci USA*, 99, 8921-6.

Kadoshima-Yamaoka, K., Murakawa, M., Goto, M., Tanaka, Y., Inoue, H., Murafuji, H., Nagahira, A., Hayashi, Y., Kagahira, K., Miura, K., Nakatsuka, T., Chamoto, K., Fukuda, Y., Nishimura, T. (2009). ASB16165, a novel inhibitor for phosphodiesterase 7A (PDE7A), supresses IL-12-induced IFN-γ production by mouse activated T lymphocytes. *Immunol Letters*, 122, 193-7.

Karatza, A.A., Bush, A., Magee, A.G. (2005). Safety and efficacy of sildenafil therapy in children with pulmonary hypertension. *Int J Cardiol*, 100, 267-73.

Koike, T., Nadeen Qutab, M., Tsuchida, M., Takekubo, M., Saito, M., Hayashi, J. (2008). Pretreatment with olprinone hydrochloride, a phosphodiesterase III inhibitor, attenuates lipopolysaccharide-induced lung injury via and anti-inflammatory effect. *Pulm Pharmacol Ther*, 21, 161-77.

Korhonen, K., Kiuru, A., Svedstrom, E., Kaapa, P. (2004). Pentoxyfylline reduces regional inflammatory and ventilatory disturbances in meconium-exposed piglet lungs. *Pediatr Res*, 56, 901-6.

Lapenna, D., De Gioia, S., Mezzetti, A., Ciofani, G., Festi, D., Cuccurullo, F. (1995). Aminophylline: could it act as an antioxidant in vivo? *Eur J Clin Invest*, 25, 464-70.

Luo, W.J., Ling, X., Huang, R.M. (2004). Effects of aminophylline on cytokines and pulmonary functions undergoing valve replacement. *Eur J Cardiothorac Surg*, 25, 766-71.

Mascali, J.J., Cvietusa, P., Negri, J., Borish, L. (1996). Anti-inflammatory effects of theophylline: modulation of cytokine production. *Ann Allergy Asthma Immunol*, 77, 34-8.

Matera, M.G., Page, C.P., Cazzola, M. (2011). Novel bronchodilators for the treatment of chronic obstructive pulmonary disease. *Trends in Pharmacol Sci*, 32, 495-506.

Minton, N.A., Henry, J.A. (1996). Acute and chronic human toxicity of theophylline. *Hum Exp Toxicol*, 15, 471-81.

Mokra, D., Drgova, A., Mokry, J., Bulikova, J., Pullmann, R., Durdik, P., Petraskova, M., Calkovska, A. (2008a). Combination of budesonide and aminophylline diminished acute lung injury in animal model of meconium aspiration syndrome. *J Physiol Pharmacol*, 59, 461-71.

Mokra, D., Drgova, A., Mokry, J., Pullmann, R., Redfors, B., Petraskova, M., Calkovska, A. (2008b). Comparison of the effects of low-dose vs. high-dose aminophylline on lung function in experimental meconium aspiration syndrome. *J Physiol Pharmacol*, 59, 449-59.

Mokra, D., Drgova, A., Pullmann, R. Sr, Calkovska, A. (2012). Selective phosphodiesterase 3 inhibitor olprinone attenuates meconium-induced oxidative lung injury. *Pulm Pharmacol Ther*, 25, 216-22.

Mokra, D., Mokry, J. (2007). Inflammation in meconium aspiration syndrome: targets for pharmacological modulation. *Current Pediatr Rev*, 3, 248-63.

Mokra, D., Mokry, J. (2010). *Meconium Aspiration Syndrome: From Pathomechanisms to Treatment* (1st edition). New York, USA: Nova Biomedical Books.

Mokra, D., Mokry, J., Tatarkova, Z., Redfors, B., Petraskova, M., Calkovska, A. (2007). Aminophylline treatment in meconium-induced acute lung injury in a rabbit model. *J Physiol Pharmacol*, 58, 399-407.

Mokra, D., Tonhajzerova, I., Mokry, J., Petraskova, M., Hutko, M., Calkovska, A. (2013). Cardiovascular side effects of aminophylline in meconium-induced acute lung injury. *Adv Exp Med Biol*, 756, 341-7.

Mokry, J., Mokra, D. (2013). Immunological aspects of phosphodiesterase inhibition in the respiratory system. *Respir Physiol Neurobiol*, in press.

Mokry, J., Mokra, D., Nosalova, G., Beharkova, M., Feherova, Z. (2008). Influence of selective inhibitors of phosphodiesterase 3 and 4 on cough and airway reactivity. *J Physiol Pharmacol*, 59, 473-82.

Mokry, J., Nosalova, G. (2011). The influence of the PDE inhibitors on cough reflex in guinea pigs. *Bratisl Lek Listy*, 112(3), 131-5

Mokry, J., Nosalova, G., Mokra, D. (2009). Influence of xanthine derivatives on cough and airway reactivity in guinea pigs. *J Physiol Pharmacol*, 60, 87-91.

Morales-Garcia, J.A., Redondo, M., Alonso-Gil, S., Gil, C., Perez, C., Martinez, A., Santos, A., Perez-Castillo, A. (2011). Phosphodiesterase 7 Inhibition Preserves Dopaminergic Neurons in Cellular and Rodent Models of Parkinson Disease. *PLoS ONE*, 6, e17240.

Nakata, A., Ogawa, K., Sasaki, T., Koyama, N., Wada, K., Kotera, J., Kokkawa, H., Omori, K., Kaminuma, O. (2002). Potential role of phosphodiesterase 7 in human T cell function: comparative effects of two phosphodiesterase inhibitors. *Clin Exp Immunol*, 128, 460-6.

Nosalova, G, Mokry, J. (2001). The mechanism of action of xanthine derivatives and suppression of cough. *Acta Med Mart*, 1, 14-8.

Nosalova, G. (2000). New opinions on the mechanism of action of xanthine derivatives. *Slovakofarma Revue*, 10, 51-5.

Paterniti, I., Mazzon, E., Gil, C., Impellizzeri, D., Palomo, V., Redondo, M., Perez, D.I., Esposito, E., Martinez, A., Cuzzocrea, S. (2011). PDE7 inhibitors: new potential drugs for the therapy of spinal cord injury. *PLoS ONE*, 6, e15937.

Peters-Golden, M., Canetti, C., Mancuso, P., Coffey, M.J. (2005). Leukotrienes: underappreciated mediators of innate immune responses. *J Immunol*, 174, 589–94.

Pitts, W.J., Vaccaro, W., Huynh, T., Leftheris, K., Roberge, J.Y., Barbosa, J., Guo, J., Brown, B., Watson, A., Donaldson, K., Starling, G.C., Kiener, P.A., Poss, M.A., Dodd, J.H., Barrish, J.C. (2004). Identification of purine inhibitors of phosphodiesterase 7 (PDE7). *Bioorganic Medicinal Chemistry Letters*, 14, 2955-8.

Polson, J.B., Kazanowski J.J., Goildman A.L., Szentivanyi A. (1978). Inhibition of human pulmonary phosphodiesterase activity by therapeutic levels of theophylline. *Clin Exp Phramacol Physiol*, 5, 535-9.

Rabe, K.F., Bateman, E.D., O`Donnell, D., Witte, S., Bredenbroker, D., Bethke, T.D. (2005). Roflumilast – an oral anti-inflammatory treatment for chronic obstructive pulmonary disease: a randomised controlled trial. *Lancet*, 366, 563-71.

Rabe, K.F., Magnussen, H., Dent, G. (1995). Theophylline and selective PDE inhibitors as bronchodilators and smooth muscle relaxants. *Eur Respir J*, 8, 637-42.

Rennard, S., Knobil, K., Rabe, K.F., Morris, A., Schachter, N., Locantore, N., Canonica, W.G., Zhu, Y., Barnhart, F. (2008). The efficacy and safety of cilomilast in COPD. *Drugs*, 68, 3-57.

Roberts, G., Newsom, D., Gomez, K. on behalf of the North West Thames Asthma Study Group. (2003). Intravenous salbutamol bolus compared with an aminophylline infusion in children with severe asthma: a randomized controlled trial. *Thorax*, 58, 306-10.

Salari, P., Mojtahedzadeh, M., Najafi, A., Sadraie, S., Bahaadini, K., Moharreri, M., Hadavand, N., Abdollahi, M. (2005). Comparison of the effect of aminophylline and low PEEP vs. high PEEP on EGF concentration in critically ill patients with ALI/ARDS. *J Clin Pharmacy Therapeutics*, 30, 139-44.

Sanz, M.J., Cortijo, J., Morcillo, E.J. (2005). PDE4 inhibitors as new antiinflammatory drugs: effects on cell trafficking and cell adhesion molecules expression. *Pharmacol Ther*, 106, 269-297.

Sastry, B.K., Narasimhan, C., Reddy, N.K., Raju, B.S. (2004). Clinical efficacy of sildenafil in primary pulmonary hypertension: a randomized, placebo-controlled, double-blind, crossover study. *J Am Coll Cardiol*, 43, 1149-53.

Sebkhi, A., Strange, J.W., Phillips, S.C., Wharton, J., Wilkins, M.R. (2003). Phosphodiesterase type 5 as a target for the treatment of hypoxia-induced pulmonary hypertension. *Circulation*, 107, 3230-5.

Shakur, Y., Holst, L.S., Landstrom, T.R., Movesian, M., Degerman, E., Manganiello, V. (2001). Regulation and function of the cyclic nucleotide phosphodiesterase (PDE3) gene family. *Prog Nucleic Acid Res Mol Biol*, 66, 241-77.

Shekerdemian, L.S., Ravn, H.B., Penny, D.J. (2002). Intravenous sildenafil lowers pulmonary vascular resistance in a model of neonatal pulmonary hypertension. *Am J Respir Crit Care Med*, 165, 1098-102.

Smith, S.J., Brookes-Fazakerley, S., Donnelly, L.E., Barnes, P.J., Barnette, M.S., Giembycz, M.A. (2003). Ubiquitous expression of phosphodiesterase 7A in human proinflammatory and immune cells. *Am J Physiol Lung Cell Mol Physiol*, 284, L279-89.

Smith, S.J., Cieslinski, L.B., Newton, R., Donnelly, L.E., Fenwick, P.S., Nicholson, A.G., Barnes, P.J., Barnette, M.S., Giembycz, M.A. (2004). Discovery of BRL 50481 [3-(N,N-dimethylsulfonamido)-4-methylnitrobenzene], a Selective Inhibitor of Phosphodiesterase 7: In Vitro Studies in Human Monocytes, Lung Macrophages, and CD8+ TLymphocytes. *Molecular Pharmacology*, 66, 1679-1689.

Spicuzza, L., Di Maria, G., Polosa, R. (2006). Adenosine in the airways: Implications and applications. *Eur J Pharmacol*, 533, 77-88.

Spina, D. (2008). PDE4 inhibitors: current sttus. *Br J Pharmacol*, 155, 308-15.

Tegtmeyer, F.K., Heilemann, A., Reiss, I., Fischer, T. (2002). Inhibition of meconium induced activation of granulocytes from neonates and adults by pentoxyphylline. *Klin Pädiatr*, 214, 347-52.

Toward, T.J., Smith, N., Broadley, K.J. (2004). Effect of phosphodiesterase-5 inhibitor, sildenafil (Viagra), in animal models of irways disease. *Am J Respir Crit Care Med*, 169, 227-34.

Vestbo, J., Tan, L., Atkinson, G., Ward J on behalf of the UK-500,001 Global Study Team. (2009). A controlled trial of 6-weeks` treatment with a novel inhaled phosphodiesterase type-4 inhibitor in COPD. *Eur Respir J*, 33, 1039-44.

Wang, Y.J., Jiang, Y.L., Tang, H.F., Zhao, C.Z., Chen, J.Q. (2010). Zl-n-91, a selective phosphodiesterase 4 inhibitor, supresses inflammatory response in a COPD-like rat model. *Int Immunopharmacol*, 10, 252-8.

Wharton, J., Strange, J.W., Moller, G.M., Growcott, E.J., Ren, X., Franklyn, A.P., Phillips, S.C., Wilkins, M.R. (2005). Antiproliferative effects of phosphodiesterase type 5 inhibition in human pulmonary artery cells. *Am J Respir Crit Care Med*, 172, 105-13.

Yamamoto, S., Sugahara, S., Ikeda, K., Shimizu, Y. (2006). Pharmacological profile of a novel phosphodiesterase 7A and -4 dual inhibitor, YM-393059, on acute and chronic inflammation models. *Eur J Pharmacol*, 550, 166-72.

Zheng, H., Crowley, J.J., Chan, J.C., Hoffmann, H., Hatherill, J.R., Ishizaka, A., Raffin, T.A. (1990). Attenuation of tumor necrosis factor-induced endothelial cell cytotoxicity and neutrophil chemiluminescence. *Am Rev Respir Dis*, 142, 1073-8.

Reviewed by:

Martin Wawruch, MD., PhD., Assoc. Prof., Department of Pharmacology and Clinical Pharmacology, Faculty of Medicine, Comenius University, Bratislava, Slovakia;

Jana Plevkova, MD., PhD., Assoc. Prof., Department of Pathological Physiology, Jessenius Faculty of Medicine, Comenius University, Martin, Slovakia.

In: Neonatal Care: New Research
Editors: F. Koubek and J. Linser
ISBN: 978-1-62618-454-1

Chapter 3

Glucocorticoids in Meconium Aspiration Syndrome: Possible Benefits Versus Risks of the Treatment

Daniela Mokra[1,*] and Juraj Mokry[2†]
[1]Department of Physiology,
[2]Department of Pharmacology,
Jessenius Faculty of Medicine, Comenius University, Martin, Slovakia

Abstract

Glucocorticoids possess a lot of pharmacological properties useful in the treatment of various diseases. In meconium aspiration syndrome (MAS), a serious neonatal disease with complex pathophysiology, glucocorticoids have been administered in experimental and clinical studies with more or less success according to design of the study, type of glucocorticoid derivative, dose and mode of delivery. Nevertheless, despite growing information on positive effects of glucocorticoid treatment on the lung edema, inflammation and pulmonary vasoconstriction, many questions have not been answered yet, e.g. on

* Corresponding author: Daniela Mokra, MD., PhD. Department of Physiology, Jessenius Faculty of Medicine, Comenius University. Mala Hora 4, 03601 Martin, Slovakia. Phone: +421 432633454. E-mail: mokra@jfmed.uniba.sk.

† E-mail: mokry@jfmed.uniba.sk.

possible side effects of the treatment. To consider objectively the positives and negatives of the glucocorticoid administration in MAS, this chapter reviews the pathomechanims of MAS, mechanisms of action of glucocorticoids, as well as effects of various glucocorticoids delivered in experimental models and in newborns with MAS.

Keywords: Glucocorticoids, meconium aspiration syndrome, animal model, newborn

ABBREVIATIONS

ANP:	atrial natriuretic peptide
AP-1:	protein activator-1
cGR:	cytoplasmic GC receptor
COX:	cyclooxygenase
ET-1:	endothelin 1
GC:	glucocorticoid
GCs:	glucocorticoids
GM-CSF:	granulocyte-monocyte colony stimulating factor
11β-HSD:	11β-hydroxysteroid dehydrogenase
HSP90:	heat shock protein 90
GR:	glucocorticoid receptor
mGR:	membrane-bound GC receptor
GRE:	glucocorticoid responsive element
ICAM:	intercellular adhesion molecule
IL:	interleukin
iNOS:	inducible NO synthase
LPS:	lipopolysaccharide
MAPK:	mitogen activated protein kinase
MR:	mineralocorticoid receptor
NFκB:	nuclear factor κB
PG:	prostaglandin
PAF:	platelet activating factor
PLA_2:	phospholipase A_2
RONS:	reactive oxygen and nitrogen species
SLPI:	secretory leukocyte proteinase inhibitor
TGFβ:	transforming growth factor β
TNFα:	tumor necrosis factor α.

INTRODUCTION

Meconium Aspiration Syndrome (MAS)

Meconium aspiration syndrome (MAS) is a major cause of respiratory insufficiency in the term and post-term newborns. Incidence of MAS in the developed countries stands about 1-2 per 1000 live births, but in the developing countries and in subpopulations with lower social standards this number may be higher (Dargaville et al. 2006). Clinical signs of the disorder vary from mild tachypnoea to severe respiratory failure associated with pulmonary hypertension (Co and Vidyasagar 1990). In addition to acute effects, MAS may cause also serious long-term consequences on the respiratory system, whereas abnormal bronchial reactivity, wheezing and other respiratory pathology were found in a portion of infants who overcome MAS in the neonatal period (Vázquez Nava et al. 2006).

Because of complex pathogenesis of the disease and multiple interactions between the individual pathomechanisms, treatment of MAS is still problematic. In the last years, many adjunctive or alternative approaches have been tested in MAS. Since some of them have been rather well established (e.g. different modes of ventilatory support, surfactant administration or inhaled nitric oxide), therapeutic potential of others (particularly of anti-inflammatory drugs and vasodilators) is under research (Mokra and Mokry 2010).

PATHOGENESIS OF MAS AS A RATIONALE FOR THE TREATMENT BY GLUCOCORTICOIDS

Airway Obstruction

In an acute phase of the disease, aspirated meconium may obstruct the airways. Complete airway obstruction by thick meconium results in alveolar atelectasis behind the plug. Furthermore, perfusion of non-ventilated alveoli increases the right-to-left pulmonary shunts and in severe cases the return to a fetal type of circulation may be observed. Partial airway obstruction causes a ball-valve effect, with air-trapping and risk of air leak into the interstitium (Tyler et al. 1978).

Inflammation

With initiation of ventilation, aspirated meconium reaches the alveoli, where triggers inflammation (Wu et al. 1999). Meconium itself acts as a potent chemoattractant for neutrophils (Yamada et al. 2000) increasing their number in the lungs within several hours after the aspiration, what is linked with their decrease in the blood (Soukka et al. 1997, Mokry et al. 2006).

In addition, meconium is a source of pro-inflammatory mediators, such as interleukins (IL) -1, -6, and -8, tumor necrosis factor (TNF)α etc. (de Beaufort et al. 2003). Thus, it may induce inflammation directly or indirectly through the stimulation of oxidative burst in neutrophils (Soukka et al. 2002) and alveolar macrophages (Craig et al. 2005). Activated macrophages and released cytokines stimulate adhesion of neutrophils on the endothelium and formation the microemboli in the capillary bed, participating in the onset of pulmonary hypertension.

This process is facilitated by a complement, activation of which has been proven also in MAS (Castellheim et al. 2005). Activated cells (leukocytes, platelets, epithelial and endothelial cells etc.) produce a wide spectrum of substances, such as TNFα, IL, leukotrienes (LT), prostaglandins (PG), platelet activating factor (PAF), proteolytic enzymes, and reactive oxygen and nitrogen species (RONS), injuring the lung parenchyma and surfactant. Inflammatory cytokines induce expression of angiotensin II (ANG II), which causes apoptotic death of the lung cells after its binding to AT1 receptors, as well (Vidyasagar and Zagariya 2008). Subsequently, a leak of proteinaceous fluid and cells into the alveolar spaces through the alveolar capillary membrane further deteriorate the lung function.

Meconium contains high concentrations of phospholipase A_2 (PLA_2), which may directly or via the arachidonic acid metabolism increase the production of lipid mediators and participate in the apoptosis of epithelial cells (Holopainen et al. 1999) and surfactant dysfunction (Schrama et al. 2001). In addition, meconium enhances the expression of inducible cyclooxygenase-2 (COX-2) and inducible nitric oxide synthase (iNOS) in the macrophages, epithelial and endothelial cells (Li et al. 2001, Kytola et al. 2003). Furthermore, release of bronchoactive substances such as LT and PAF is probably responsible for increased airway reactivity to bronchoconstriction agents (Khan et al. 2002, Mokry et al. 2006).

Surfactant Dysfunction in MAS

In addition to inflammation, meconium inactivates function of pulmonary surfactant by several distinct mechanisms. Meconium:

1. slows down the adsorption of surfactant lipids and reduces the spread of surfactant film at the air: liquid interphase in the alveoli (Sun et al. 1993, Pallem et al. 2010);
2. changes the viscosity and ultrastructure of surfactant (Bae et al. 1998, Pallem et al. 2010);
3. decreases the levels of surfactant proteins (Cleary et al. 1997); and
4. accelerates the conversion from large, surface active surfactant aggregates into small, less active forms (Kakinuma et al. 2002, Ochs et al. 2006).

Components of meconium (cholesterol, free fatty acids, bile acids, lysophospholipids, bilirubin etc.) interfere with surfactant ability to reduce the surface tension at air: liquid interphase during compression of the surface and fluidize the surfactant film (Diemel et al. 2002, Zuo et al. 2008). In addition, bile acids penetrate through the lamellar structures and surfactant monolayer and alleviate a leak of cholesterol into the surfactant complexes and further injure their function (Lopez-Rodriguez et al. 2011). High concentrations of bile acids increase the production and activation of phospholipase A_2 in the lungs. PLA_2 then directly or indirectly through its products, such as lysophosholipids, affects the surfactant metabolism and damages the cell membranes, as well (De Luca et al. 2011).

Dysfunction of surfactant is potentiated by plasma proteins leaking through an injured alveolar capillary membrane. Plasma proteins may deteriorate surfactant function via different mechanisms. Albumin, fibrinogen and hemoglobin inhibit the surfactant through competitive adsorption with surfactant phospholipids at an air: liquid interphase (Holm et al. 1999). Furthermore, albumin interacts with double-layer of phospholipids and thereby interrupts their distribution in the structures of surfactant (Larsson et al. 2006), and C-reactive protein fluidizes the surfactant film (Sáenz et al. 2010).

Pulmonary surfactant may be inactivated also by the action of proteolytic enzymes and RONS released from activated cells during the inflammation. For example, TNFα and IL-1 inhibit expression of surfactant proteins (Hallman et al., 2001), and RONS damage both the surfactant proteins and phospholipids (Rodríguez-Capote et al. 2006). Structure and function of surfactant may be enzymatically degradated by proteolytic enzymes including phospholipase A_2, as well (De Luca et al. 2011).

Pulmonary Vasoconstriction in MAS

Meconium aspiration is often associated with pulmonary vasoconstriction from hypoxia and/or from vasoconstriction effect of meconium and substances released during the inflammation. Presence of meconium in the fetal amniotic fluid may cause ischemic changes of the lungs, umbilical cord, and placenta (Burgess and Hutchins 1996). Postnatal meconium instillation elevates the pulmonary artery pressure and vascular resistance in a concentration-dependent manner (Holopainen et al. 1998), what is linked with higher levels of thromboxane A_2 (TXA_2), LT, PG, and endothelin-1 (ET-1) (Soukka et al. 1998b, Kuo and Chen 1999, Wu et al. 1999).

Glucocorticoids (GCs)

Mechanisms of Action

GCs play a fundamental role in the response to stress including trauma, sepsis, starvation and tissue ischaemia, as well as to psychological stress. Such stimulation activates the hypothalamic-pituitary-adrenal (HPA) axis and results in increased release of cortisol. Cortisol induces adaptive responses that may be homeostatic (adjusting systems to function normally in the stressful situation) or allostatic (adjusting systems to function in a manner more appropriate to the stressful environment). GCs provide a brake on innate inflammatory mechanisms, promoting resolution of inflammation. GCs reduce penetration of neutrophils into the lungs decreasing their adherence to the endothelium and thereby increase secondarily count of circulating neutrophils (Soukka et al. 1997, Holopainen et al. 2001, Mokra et al. 2007a, Mokra et al. 2007b). Moreover, GCs decrease counts of circulating mononuclears, eosinophils, and basophils as well as synthesis of cytokines by macrophages, eosinophils, and T-lymphocytes. GCs stabilize lysosomes, inhibit release of lysosomal enzymes, chemotaxia and other functions of neutrophils, as well (Jantz and Sahn 1999). Stabilizing the cell membranes and decreasing production of pro-inflammatory and vasoactive substances GCs reduce microvascular permeability. In addition, by direct modulation of the pulmonary vasomotoric tone GCs diminish pulmonary vasoconstriction and inhibit fibrogenesis (Jantz and Sahn, 1999, Fernandes et al. 2005, Czock et al. 2005). However, GCs affect also the cardiovascular system and metabolism, e.g. keeping the blood pressure and recruiting glucose to supply energy in a stressful situation (Sapolsky et al. 2000, Lee et al. in press).

Secretion of cortisol in the adrenal cortex is controlled by free cortisol level in the plasma, the sleep-wake cycle and corticotrophin-releasing hormone. Cortisol mediates its effects via activation of intracellular glucocorticoid receptors (GR or low affinity receptors), which are expressed ubiquitously (Walker 2007). In addition, cortisol interacts with mineralocorticoid receptors (MR or high affinity receptors), which are expressed only in selected tissues and at lower levels. In some tissues (distal nephron, salivary and sweat glands, vascular endothelium etc.), MRs bind exclusively aldosterone, as cortisol is excluded by local pre-receptor inactivation by 11β-hydroxysteroid dehydrogenase type 2 (HSD2) to inert cortisone. Contrary in myocardium, vascular smooth muscle or adipose tissue, MRs are occupied by cortisol in competition with much lower prevailing concentrations of aldosterone and active cortisol regenerates from inactive cortisone under the influence of 11β-HSD1 amplifying GR activation (Tomlinson et al. 2004, Walker 2007). The mentioned intracellular MRs and GCs receptors act as transcription factors on approximately one third of genes, as the pattern of response in individual cell types depends on the complexity of interactions with heterodimers, co-activators and co-repressors, and epigenetic factors including chromatin organisation (Walker 2007). Thus, also the effect of synthetic steroids varies according to their susceptibility to metabolism by 11β-HSDs and binding affinity for GR and MR. For example, dexamethasone is relatively resistant to 11β-HSDs and acts as potent selective GR agonist, but prednisolone is relatively selective for GR over MR and is susceptible to metabolism by 11β-HSDs (Diederich et al. 2004).

In immune cells, expression of 11β-HSD enzymes is not completely understood. In *in vitro* studies, 11β-HSD1 was expressed upon differentiation of human monocytes to macrophages, while 11β-HSD2 was not detectable in either monocytes or cultured macrophages. Several cytokines, such as IL-4 and IL-13, up-regulate an expression of 11β-HSD1, what may result in increased level of active intracellular cortisol and suppressed production of inflammatory mediators by macrophages (Thieringer et al. 2001). On the other hand, TNFα, IL-1β, LPS, or IL-6 failed to increase the 11β-HSD1 activity in the monocytes, but TNFα and IL-1β induced 11β-HSD1 activity in human aortic and bronchial smooth muscle cells (Cai et al. 2001).

Thus, 11β-HSD1 functions as a reductase converting inactive cortisone to the active cortisol in cells. Cortisol and other GCs mediate most of their effects *genomically* by binding to glucocorticoid receptor (GR) that results in the *transactivation* of genes controlled by glucocorticoid response elements (GRE) and induction (or "switching-on") of anti-inflammatory genes expression. This mechanism directly modulates the expression of anti-inflammatory cytokines IL-10 and TGFβ, secretory leukocyte proteinase inhibitor (SLPI), IL-1 receptor antagonist or C1q, as well as annexin 1 (or lipocortin 1) mediating many of the anti-inflammatory actions of GCs (Barnes 1998, Czock et al. 2005, McColl et al. 2007). Nevertheless, most of genes are regulated indirectly by the GR via suppression of gene expression (or *transrepression*). Ligand-activated GR can "switch-off" expression of the inflammatory genes through protein-protein interactions with activated NFκB and AP-1 transcription factors, finally leading to suppressed synthesis of pro-inflammatory substances, such as cytokines (IL-1, IL-2, IL-6, IL-12, TNFα, GM-CSF), chemokines (IL-8, eotaxin, MIP-1α), proinflammatory enzymes (COX-2, $cPLA_2$, iNOS) or adhesion molecules (ICAM-1, E-selectin) (Czock et al. 2005, McColl et al. 2007). As higher concentrations of GCs are required for induction of anti-inflammatory gene expression than for gene repression, repression of pro-inflammatory transcription factors appears to be the dominant mechanism of GC action (McColl et al. 2007). However, there is an additional DNA binding-independent mechanism of GCs action – reversible alterations in chromatin structure and histone acetylation. This process may be important for "switching-off" genes once the stimulus is removed and inflammation is no longer required (McColl et al. 2007).

In the mentioned genomically-mediated processes, transcription and translation with subsequent proteosynthesis require at least 30 min up to several hours/days until some changes may be observed (Goulding 2004). However, GCs act also through *nongenomically-mediated mechanisms*, which are responsible for rapid GCs action (within seconds to minutes) until the effects mediated by genomic mechanisms occure (Stellato 2004). In literature, several possible nongenomic mechanisms are discussed, such as specific interaction with the cytosolic GR receptor and successive release of HSP-90 and special proteins Src and MAPK, or specific interactions with membrane-bound glucocorticoid receptors (Buttgereit and Scheffold 2002). However, some immediate GCs effects may be GR independent, e.g. inhibition of superoxide production by macrophages (Long et al. 2005)] or interactions with cell membranes (Buttgereit and Scheffold 2002). GCs may exert rapid effects on various tissues and cells modulating hormone secretion, neuronal excitability, carbohydrate metabolism, cell morphology, cell behaviour, and other processes within seconds or minutes (Falkenstein et al. 2000, Stellato 2004). The GCs may nongenomically affect ion cycling (Verriére et al. 2005), cellular energy metabolism (Buttgereit and Scheffold 2002), or neuronal activity (Chen and Qiu 2001), as well as the second messenger systems (Buttgereit and Scheffold 2002). In respiratory system, GCs may modulate Na^+/H^+ exchange activity in bronchial epithelial cells (Verriére et al. 2005) and inhibit airway smooth muscle contraction, as was observed within 10 min after GCs inhalation (Zhou et al. 2003, Sun et al. 2006). Similarly, in a rabbit model of MAS GCs significantly improved several respiratory parameters already within 30 min after the administration (Mokra et al. 2007b, Mokra et al. 2007c).

Interactions between genomic and nongenomic mechanisms have been claimed, thereby controlling genomic mechanisms through nongenomic ones (Wehling 1997). Nongenomic effects occur faster and may be clinically relevant over a limited period "bridging the gap" until the genomic effects take place (Buttgereit et al. 1999).

Irrespective of mechanisms of their action, GCs effectively suppress inflammation, lung edema formation, and pulmonary vasoconstriction. In addition, GCs act as important regulators of apoptosis and phagocytic removal of apoptotic cells, and thereby influence resolution of inflammation (McColl et al. 2007). GCs may have apoptotic or antiapoptotic effects, depending on the cell type. For example, GCs increase the rate of apoptosis in eosinophils, what might be important in attenuation of the inflammatory response e.g. in asthma. On the other hand, GCs decrease the rate of apoptosis in neutrophils what might explain a limited efficacy of GCs in chronic bronchopulmonary disease (COPD), where the neutrophilic inflammation prevails (Czock et al. 2005)].

Side Effects of GCs

As stress hormones, GCs released via the hypothalamic-pituitary-adrenal axis recruit glucose to supply energy to organs facing stress, leading to arousal reactions and immune responses to maintain homeostasis. Failure to keep ample concentrations of GCs adversely affects metabolism and organ function (Lee et al. in press).

GCs oppose the effects of insulin and increase turnover between the stored energy (in glycogen, triglycerides and protein) and freely available fuel for mitochondrial oxidation (glucose and free fatty acids) (Walker 2007). Long-term stimulation or administration of excessive GCs may then result in various pathological manifestations, such as protein catabolism, gluconeogenesis and glucogenesis resulting in hyperglycemia, and other changes such as hypokalemia, dyslipidemia, reduced fibrinolysis, posterior subcapsular cataract, exacerbation of glaucoma, increased intracranial pressure, peptic ulcers, upper gastrointestinal bleeding, immunosuppression, neuropsychiatric disturbances, osteoporosis, myopathy, irregularities of the menstruation cycle etc. (Jantz and Sahn, 1999, Schäcke et al. 2002, Fernandes et al. 2005).

GCs affect also the cardiovascular parameters. GCs raise the blood pressure, only in part mediated by renal sodium retention and plasma volume expansion (Whitworth et al. 2000). In addition, both GR and MR receptors are expressed in cardiovascular tissues including the heart and arterial walls, where GCs act directly to maintain vascular tone and modify vascular inflammatory, proliferative and remodelling responses to injury (Ullian 1999, Walker 2007).

Due to wide spectrum of side effects of systemic GCs, local administration of GCs is preferred if possible. However, dependently on the delivery system and the dose, <20% of the nebulized GCs is deposited into the lungs and the rest may be absorbed into the circulation and cause systemic effects (Rizzo and Solé 2006).

In addition, inhalation of GCs may worsen the local immunity and increase the risk of oropharyngeal candidosis, dysphonia, cough, throat irritation and other local side effects (Barnes 1995).

Nevertheless, adverse effects of GCs appear more likely after the long-term treatment, but less-frequently after the short-term treatment, even with high GCs doses. It might be explained by time-dependent genomic effects of GCs, which do not elevate further after high doses, when GR saturation is already achieved (Frauman 1996, Czock et al. 2005). Because in MAS high-dose GCs are administered in single or just several doses, some acute adverse effects, particularly cardiovascular might be expected with minimum effects e.g. on the metabolism.

Glucocorticoids in the Treatment of MAS

Effect of the treatment depends on the specific pharmacological properties, dose, and mode of delivery of the individual GCs as well as on current status of the newborn or experimental animal with MAS, concomittant diseases etc. Different properties of individual GCs are related to different mineralocorticoid activity and potency to suppress cortisol production, as well as to the potency of their nongenomic action. For example, the potency of dexamethasone was superior to other tested GCs, probably thanks to the lowest lipophilicity, that enables direct interaction with the cell membrane (Buttgereit et al. 1999, Lösel and Wehling 2003).

Several GC preparations - hydrocortisone, prednisolone, methylprednisolone, dexamethasone and budesonide - have been used in animal models and in newborns with MAS.

Anti-inflammatory effect of *hydrocortisone*, a synthetic equivalent of cortisol, is rather low compared to other synthetic GCs, i.e. 4-times lower than prednisolone and 30-times lower than dexamethasone. In addition, due to interaction with both GR and MR receptors, hydrocortisone may potentiate a disbalance of liquid and electrolytes in the body. In newborn rabbits, subcutaneous hydrocortisone at a dose of 7.5 mg/kg immediately after the meconium instillation and then every 8 hours up to 48 hours non-significantly improved histology of the lungs and decreased frequency of breathing. However, higher mortality of the hydrocortisone-treated animals was observed irrespective they aspired meconium or saline, probably due to infection at the tracheotomy site and sepsis (Frantz et al. 1975). In the study by Yeh et al. (1977), hydrocortisone at a dose of 20 mg/kg was administered 4-times every 12 hours via umbilical catheter in 17 neonates with MAS. Blood gases, x-ray, incidence of pneumothorax or pneumomediastinum, requirements for mechanical ventilation and mortality were similar in the hydrocortisone-treated vs. placebo-administered group. However, longer period to wean to room air and persisted signs of respiratory distress were observed in the treated group than in controls (Yeh et al. 1977). No benefit of the treatment might be attributed to low dose and/or late administration of the treatment, as well as to weak anti-inflammatory potential and to fluid retention in the lungs or delayed reabsorption of the fluid due to mineralocorticoid action of hydrocortisone.

Prednisolone possess predominant glucocorticoid and low mineralocorticoid activity. Intravenous administration of prednisolone at standard (2 mg/kg) and high (30 mg/kg) dose immediately after the meconium instillation enhanced gas exchange and increased frequency of breathing in meconium-instilled puppies in comparison with non-treated group. Furthermore, high-dose prednisolone showed more obvious improvement in lung histology compared to the standard-dose one, without hyperglycemia or hypertension observed as side effects. Nevertheless, high-dose prednisolone paradoxically potentiated oxidation stress, indicated by elevated plasma levels of malonyldialdehyde compared to the standard-dose group and controls at 20 hours after meconium aspiration (Kirimi et al. 2003).

Methylprednisolone, a methylated derivative of prednisolone, has similar properties as prednisolone. In a porcine model of MAS, pretreatment with methylprednisolone (30 mg/kg i.v.) 30 min. before instillation of meconium tended to prevent an early (0-1 h) increase in pulmonary artery pressure and inhibited significantly the second phase (1-6 h) progressive rise in pulmonary artery pressure and pulmonary vascular resistance, decreased venous admixture and formation of lung edema and improved oxygenation (Soukka et al. 1997). In addition, premedication with methylprednisolone decreased endothelin (ET)-1 and increased atrial natriuretic peptide (ANP). Modulation of the ratio ET-1/ANP for ANP reduced pulmonary hypertension and indicated protective effect of GCs on the endothelium-mediated regulation of the pulmonary vascular tone (Soukka et al. 1998a). Thus, premedication with GCs before the labour might be beneficial in case of verified massive meconium staining of the amniotic fluid and prenatal meconium aspiration to reduce remodelling of the pulmonary vascular bed and lung inflammation. However, up to this time no clinical study was performed to evaluate possible benefits of prenatal GCs delivery in MAS. In the clinical trial by Basu et al. (2007), methylprednisolone administered for a period of 7 days starting after 24 h of age in 34 newborns with MAS shortened a period of oxygen delivery and duration of hospital stay and improved radiological clearance of the lungs, while no serious adverse effects were observed. In the study by Tripathi and co-workers (Tripathi and Saili 2007, Tripathi et al. 2007)], methylprednisolone was given in 17 newborns with MAS at a dose of 0.5 mg/kg/day i.v. in two divided doses every 12 hours for 7 days. Methylprednisolone treatment shortened duration of stay, oxygen dependence and x-ray of the lungs, decreased levels of TNFα in tracheal aspirate and did not increase incidence of sepsis.

Dexamethasone has potent anti-inflammatory and immunosuppressive effects. It is about 30-times stronger than hydrocortisone and about 5-times stronger than prednisone. In newborns with severe MAS, dexamethasone stabilized cardiovascular parameters, improved lung functions and facilitated weaning from the ventilator (Wu et al. 1999). Later, many experimental and clinical studies evaluated efficacy and management of dexamethasone delivery in the conditions of MAS. Commonly, a dose of 0.5 mg/kg body weight of dexamethasone has been established. Nevertheless, timing of dexamethasone administration appeared to be critical for effectiveness of the treatment. Pretreatment with dexamethasone (1 hour before meconium instillation) reduced pulmonary vascular resistance and lung edema, improved oxygenation and prevented ultrastructural changes of the lungs in meconium-instilled piglets (Holopainen et al. 2001). Similarly, early administration of dexamethasone (30 min after meconium instillation) significantly improved right-to-left pulmonary shunting and gas exchange, and allowed to decrease ventilatory pressures in meconium-instilled rabbits compared to non-treated controls (Mokra et al. 2007c). In addition, early dexamethasone decreased percentage of neutrophils in the bronchoalveolar lavage fluid, diminished lung edema, meconium-induced tracheal hyperresponsiveness to histamine, and decreased concentrations of lipid and protein peroxidation products in the lung homogenate compared to non-treated controls (Mokra et al. 2007c, Mokry et al. 2006). Contrary, late administration of dexamethasone (1 hour after meconium instillation) had no significant effect on oxygenation and lung edema in piglets with MAS (Holopainen et al. 2001)]. These results have clearly showed superior effect of early administration of GCs before generation of extensive inflammatory response to the meconium instillation. Nevertheless, limitations of the treatment efficacy in the late administration of GCs may be partially reduced by repetitive administration. It is known that action of dexamethasone is fast, but short-term, with plasma half-time in adults about 190 min. Therefore, dexamethasone might be administered repetitively every 2-4 hours (data given by producer, Dexamed, Medochemie Cyprus). In meconium-instilled piglets, two-phase dexamethasone delivery at 2 and 8 hours after meconium instillation significantly enhanced gas exchange and lung compliance compared to controls (Khan et al. 1999). In a rabbit model of MAS, repetitive administration of dexamethasone 0.5 and 2.5 hours after meconium instillation suppressed inflammation and improved gas exchange more effectively than a single-dose administered 0.5 hour after meconium (Mokra et al. 2008a, Mokra et al. 2007c). In newborns with MAS, dexamethasone in gradually decreasing doses within maximally 9 days (at a dose of 0.5, 0.25, and 0.125 mg/kg/day, each dosing for 3 days) decreased oxygenation index and facilitated weaning from the ventilator (da Costa et al. 2001). Nevertheless, high doses of GCs or their repetitive administration may lead to various undesirable effects. In a rabbit model of MAS, slow intravenous administration of one dose, but especially of two doses of dexamethasone was linked with acute changes of blood pressure, heart rate, and heart rate variability within 5 h of the treatment (Mokra et al. 2008a, Mokra et al. 2008c). Detailed analysis of cardiovascular changes showed increased blood pressure, decreased heart rate, increased heart rate variability and higher occurence of cardiac arrhythmia particularly during and immediately after the dexamethasone administration, while decreased heart rate and increased heart rate variability were observed till the end of the observation period (i.e. 5 hours after the first dose of dexamethasone) (Mokra et al. 2008a, Mokra et al. 2008c). Despite the acute cardiovascular changes may be critical for neonates with meconium-induced lung injury, there is a lack of information on evaluation of adverse effects of repetitive GCs administration in neonatal MAS.

Thanks to high first-pass metabolism and local delivery, treatment with inhalational *budesonide* is associated with lower incidence of systemic side effects than in the other GCs (Barnes 1995, Hvizdos and Jarvis 2000). In meconium-instilled rabbits, budesonide (0.25 mg/kg) was administered intratracheally 30 min after meconium instillation and then 2 hours later using impulsion effect of high-frequency jet ventilation (inspiration time 20%). The treatment effectively alleviated inflammation, diminished lung edema formation and meconium-induced tracheal and lung airway hyperreactivity to histamine, improved gas exchange and decreased oxidation injury of the lungs compared to non-treated controls (Mokra et al. 2007b). Furthermore, budesonide administration was associated with negligible acute cardiovascular effects (Mokra et al. 2007a) compared to dexamethasone (Mokra et al. 2008a, Mokra et al. 2008c). In newborns with MAS, budesonide given for a period of 7 days starting after 24 h of age in 32 newborns with MAS shortened a period of oxygen delivery and duration of hospital stay and improved radiological clearance of the lungs, while no serious adverse effects were found (Basu et al. 2007). In other study (Tripathi and Saili 2007, Tripathi et al. 2007)], budesonide was administered in 17 newborns with MAS at a dose of 50 μg/kg/day i.v. in two divided doses every 12 hours for 7 days. Similarly to Basu et al. (2007), budesonide shortened duration of stay, oxygen dependence and x-ray of the lungs, decreased levels of TNFα in the tracheal aspirate and did not increase risk of sepsis.

Local administration predisposes the inhalational GCs to faster and more potent action at the site of inflammation. Thanks to high lipophility, inhalational GCs including budesonide may act directly on the cells involved in the airway inflammation including macrophages, eosinophils, T-lymphocytes and epithelial cells (Barnes 1995). For example, budesonide reduced a release of IL-8 from *in vitro* airway epithelial cells 10-times stronger than dexamethasone (Pan et al. 2006)]. It corresponds well with our findings in a rabbit model of MAS that i.t. budesonide more effectively improved gas exchange and reduced lipid and protein peroxidation in the lung tissue compared to dexamethasone. In addition, budesonide reduced both tracheal and lung hyperresponsiveness to histamine, while dexamethasone decreased only tracheal reactivity with no effect on lung tissue reactivity to histamine (Mokra et al. 2007c, Mokra et al. 2007b). Nevertheless, in the above mentioned clinical studies (Basu et al. 2007, Tripathi and Saili 2007, Tripathi et al. 2007) no differences between the methylprednisolone-treated and budesonide-treated treated groups were found. Similarly, inhaled GCs (beclomethasone) showed no advantage to intravenous GCs (dexamethasone) in the ventilator-dependent preterm newborns (Suchomski and Cummings 2002). Absence of superior action of locally administered GCs to systemic GCs in these studies may be related to high losses of nebulized material out of the lungs (Rizzo and Solé 2006). On the other hand, administration directly into the trachea may effectively improve the lung functions with minimum losts of the given drug and negligible side effects (Mokra et al. 2007a, Mokra et al. 2007b).

Intratracheal delivery of GCs into the lungs may be further enhanced by a suitable vehicle, such as exogenous surfactant. In experiments, addition of GCs to exogenous surfactant did not alter the surface properties of the surfactant and GCs were well distributed throughout the lungs with 30-60% of the delivered material detected in the lung tissue (Nimmo et al. 2002)]. In preterm infants, intratracheal instillation of a mixture of budesonide (0.25 mg/kg) and beractant every 8 hours decreased mean airway pressure, oxygenation index and PCO_2 and reduced deaths and chronic lung disease at 36th week of postconceptional age compared to the group treated solely by beractant (Yeh et al. 2008). In our recent study, budesonide (0.25 mg/kg) added to exogenous surfactant Curosurf improved the lung functions and reduced inflammation in a rabbit model of MAS more effectively than a single Curosurf. In addition, improvement in oxygenation was observed immediately after the administration and the positive effect of the combined treatment remained for a longer time, while the improvement in the lung functions after the surfactant monotherapy had slower onset and shorter duration (unpublished observation). Benefits of combined administration of GCs and exogenous surfactant over the surfactant-only therapy was referred also by other authors. Intravenous dexamethasone at a single dose of 0.5 mg/kg administered within the first 5 hours of life prior a bronchoalveolar lavage using diluted beractant (5 mg/ml) in a volume of 15 ml/kg in four aliquots improved the status of the newborns with MAS more effectively than surfactant lavage alone (Salvia-Roiges et al. 2004). Similarly, combination of dexamethasone with exogenous surfactant showed an additional improvement to surfactant-only treatment in animal models of acute lung injury, as well (Chen et al. 2001, Häfner and Germann 1999)].

Utilizing their similar or additive effects, GCs may be combined also with other medicaments, e.g. with methylxanthine derivatives such as theophylline (Ito et al. 2001), with antioxidants such as N-acetylcysteine (Jansson et al. 2005) or with β2-agonists such as terbutaline (Wang et al. 2004). In experimental model of MAS, combination of intratracheal budesonide and intravenous aminophylline improved the lung functions more effectively than aminophylline-only treatment (Mokra et al. 2008b).

Conclusion

GCs are medicaments with pleiotropic effects that are mediated by genomic and by nongenomic mechanisms. Complex pathophysiology of MAS covering inflammation, lung edema and pulmonary vasoconstriction provides a rationale for the administration of GCs also in the tretament of this serious neonatal disease. Within the last decades, GCs have been used in various experimental models as well as in newborns with MAS. Favourable results from these studies indicate that GCs may be beneficial, particularly in the severe forms of MAS. However, further research is necessary to critically evaluate appropriate dosing, timing and delivery of GCs regarding their individual properties and possible acute and long-term side effects. In addition, as the causal treatment of MAS should be multi-agent, promising combinations of GCs with other drugs, particularly with exogenous surfactant, anti-inflammatory drugs and pulmonary vasodilators, should be tested in laboratory conditions.

Acknowledgments

This work was supported by the Project "Center of Excellence for Perinatology Research CEPV1 and CEPV2", co-financed from EU sources; by the Project of Slovak Research and Development Agency APVV-435-11; and by the Projects of Ministry of Education Slovak Republic VEGA No. 1/0057/11 and No. 1/0030/11.

REFERENCES

Bae, CW; Takahashi, A; Chida, S; Sasaki, M. Morphology and function of pulmonary surfactant inhibited by meconium. *Pediatr Res,* 1998 44, 187-191.

Barnes, PJ. Inhaled glucocorticoids for asthma. *N Engl J Med,* 1995 332, 868-875.

Barnes, PJ. Anti-inflammatory actions of glucocorticoids: molecular mechanisms. *Clin Sci (Lond),* 1998 94, 557-572.

Basu, S; Kumar, A; Bhatia, BD; Satya, K; Singh, TB. Role of steroids on the clinical course and outcome of meconium aspiration syndrome-a randomized controlled trial. *J Trop Pediatr,* 2007 53, 331-337.

Burgess, AM; Hutchins GM. Inflammation of the lungs, umbilical cord and placenta associated with meconium passage in utero. Review of 123 autopsied cases. *Pathol Res Pract,* 1996 192, 1121-1128

Buttgereit, F; Brand, MD; Burmester, GR. Equivalent doses and relative drug potencies for non-genomic glucocorticoid effects: a novel glucocorticoid hierarchy. *Biochem Pharmacol* 1999 58, 363-368.

Buttgereit, F; Scheffold, A. Rapid glucocorticoid effects on immune cells. *Steroids,* 2002 67, 529-534.

Cai, TQ; Wong, B;, Mundt, SS; Thieringer, R; Wright, SD; Hermanowski-Vosatka, A. Induction of 11beta-hydroxysteroid dehydrogenase type 1 but not -2 in human aortic smooth muscle cells by inflammatory stimuli. *J Steroid Biochem Mol Biol,* 2001 77, 117-122.

Castellheim, A; Lindenskov, PH; Pharo, A; Aamodt, G; Saugstad, OD; Mollness, TE. Meconium aspiration syndrome induces complement-associated systemic inflammatory response in newborn piglets. *Scand J Immunol,* 2005 61, 217-225.

Chen, CM; Fang, CL; Chang, CH. Surfactant and corticosteroid effects on lung function in a rat model of acute lung injury. *Crit Care Med,* 2001 29, 2169-2175.

Chen, YZ; Qiu, J. Possible genomic consequence of nongenomic action of glucocorticoids in neural cells. *News Physiol Sci,* 2001 16, 292-296.

Cleary, GM; Antunes, MJ; Cieselka, DA; Higgins, ST; Spitzer, AR; Chander, A. Exudative lung injury is associated with decreased levels of surfactant proteins in a rat model of meconium aspiration. *Pediatrics,* 1997 100, 998-1003.

Co, E; Vidyasagar, D. Meconium aspiration syndrome. *Compr Ther,* 1990 16, 34-39.

Craig, S; Lopez, A; Hoskin, D; Markham, F. Meconium inhibits phagocytosis and stimulates respiratory burst in alveolar macrophages. *Pediatr Res,* 2005 57, 813-818.

Czock, D; Keller, F; Rasche, FM; Häussler, U. Pharmacokinetics and pharmacodynamics of systemically administered glucocorticoids. *Clin Pharmacokinet*, 2005 44, 61-98.

da Costa, DE; Nair, AK; Pai, MG; Al Khusaiby, SM. Steroids in full term infants with respiratory failure and pulmonary hypertension due to meconium aspiration syndrome. *Eur J Pediatr,* 2001 160, 150-153.

Dargaville, PA; Copnell, B; Australian and New Zealand Neonatal Network. The epidemiology of meconium aspiration syndrome: Incidence, risk factors, therapies, and outcome. *Pediatrics,* 2006 117, 1712-1721.

de Beaufort, AJ; Bakker, AC; van Tol, MJD; Poorthius, BJ; Schrama, AJ; Berger, HM. Meconium is a source of pro-inflammatory substances and can induce cytokine production in cultured A549 epithelial cells. *Pediatr Res,* 2003 54, 491-495.

De Luca, D; Minucci, A; Tripodi, D; Piastra, M; Pietrini, D; Zuppi, C; Conti, G; Carnielli, VP; Capoluongo, E. Role of distinct phospholipases A2 and their modulators in meconium aspiration syndrome in human neonates. *Intensive Care Med,* 2011 37, 1158-1165.

Diederich, S; Scholz, T; Eigendorff, E; Bumke-Vogt, C; Quinkler, M; Exner, P; Pfeiffer, AF; Oelkers, W; Bahr, V. Pharmacodynamics and pharmacokinetics of synthetic mineralocorticoids and glucocorticoids: receptor transactivation and prereceptor metabolism by 11beta-hydroxysteroid-dehydrogenases. *Horm Metabol Res,* 2004 36, 423-429.

Diemel, RV; Snel, MM; Van Golde, LM; Putz, G; Haagsman, HP; Batenburg, JJ. Effects of cholesterol on surface activity and surface topography of spread surfactant films. *Biochemistry,* 2002 41, 15007-15016.

Falkenstein, E; Tillmann, HC; Christ, M; Feuring, M; Wehling, M. Multiple actions of steroid hormones - a focus on rapid, nongenomic effects. *Pharmacol Rev*, 2000 52, 513-556.

Fernandes, ABS; Zin, WA; Rocco, PRM. Corticosteroids in acute respiratory distress syndrome. *Braz J Med Biol Res,* 2005 38, 147-159.

Frantz, ID; Wang, NS; Thach, BT. Experimental meconium aspiration: Effects of glucocorticoid treatment. *J Pediatr,* 1975 86, 438-441.

Frauman, AG. An overview of the adverse reactions to adrenal corticosteroids. *Adverse Drug React Toxicol Rev*, 1996 15, 203-206.

Goulding, NJ. The molecular complexity of glucocorticoid actions in inflammation - a four-ring circus. *Curr Opin Pharmacol*, 2004 4, 629-636.

Häfner, D; Germann, PG. Dexamethasone enhances the activity of rSP-C surfactant but not of exosurf in a rat model of the acute lung injury. *J Pharmacol Toxicol Methods*, 1999 42, 39-48.

Hallman, M; Glumoff, V; Rämet, M. Surfactant in respiratory distress syndrome and lung injury. *Comp Biochem Physiol A Mol Integr Physiol*, 2001 129, 287-294.

Holm, BA; Wang, Z; Notter, RH. Multiple mechanisms of lung surfactant inhibition. *Pediatr Res,* 1999 46, 85-93.

Holopainen, R; Aho, H; Laine, J; Peuravuori, H; Soukka, H; Kääpä, P. Human meconium has high phospholipase A2 activity and induces cellular injury and apoptosis in piglet lungs. *Pediatr Res,* 1999 46, 626-632.

Holopainen, R; Laine, J; Halkola, L; Aho, H; Kääpä, P. Dexamethasone treatment attenuates pulmonary injury in piglet meconium aspiration. *Pediatr Res,* 2001 49, 162-168.

Holopainen, R; Soukka, H; Halkola, L; Kääpä, P. Meconium aspiration induces a concentration-dependent pulmonary hypertensive response in newborn piglets. *Pediatr Pulmonol,* 1998 25, 107-113.

Hvizdos, KM; Jarvis, B. Budesonide inhalation suspension: a review of its use in infants, children and adults with inflammatory respiratory disorders. *Drugs*, 2000 60, 1141-1178.

Ito, K; Lim, S; Caramori, G; Cosio, B; Chung, KF; Adcock, IM; Barnes, PJ. A molecular mechanism of action of theophylline: induction of histone deacetylase activity to decrease inflammatory gene expression. *Proc Natl Acad Sci USA,* 2002 99, 8921-8926.

Jansson, AH; Eriksson, C; Wang, X. Effects of budesonide and N-acetylcysteine on acute lung hyperinflation, inflammation and injury in rats. *Vascul Pharmacol,* 2005 43, 101-111.

Jantz, MA; Sahn, AS. Corticosteroids in acute respiratory failure. *Am J Respir Crit Care Med,* 1999 160, 1079-1100.

Kakinuma, R; Shimizu, H; Ogawa, Y. Effect of meconium on the rate of in vitro subtype conversion of swine pulmonary surfactant. *Eur J Pediatr,* 2002 161, 31-36.

Khan, AM; Shabarek, FM; Kutchback, JW; Lally, KP. Effects of dexamethasone on meconium aspiration syndrome in newborn piglets. *Pediatr Res,* 1999 46, 179-183.

Khan, AM; Elidemir, O; Epstein, CE; Lally, KP; Xue, H; Blackburn, M; Larsen, GL; Colasurdo, GN. Meconium aspiration produces airway hyperresponsiveness and eosinophilic inflammation in murine model. *Am J Physiol Lung Cell Mol Physiol,* 2002 283, L785-L790.

Kirimi, E; Tuncer, O; Kosem, M; Ceylan, E; Tas, A; Tasal, I; Balahoroglu, R; Caksen, H. The effects of prednisolone and serum malondialdehyde levels in puppies with experimentally induced meconium aspiration syndrome. *J Int Med Res,* 2003 31, 113-122.

Kuo, CY; Chen, JY. Effects of meconium aspiration on plasma endothelin-1 level and pulmonary hemodynamics in a piglet model. *Biol Neonate,* 1999 76, 228-234.

Kytola, J; Kääpä, P; Uotila, P. Meconium aspiration stimulates cyclooxygenase-2 and nitric oxide synthase-2 expression in rat lungs. *Pediatr Res,* 2003 53, 731-736.

Larsson, M; Nylander, T; Keough, KM; Nag, K. An X-ray diffraction study of alterations in bovine lung surfactant bilayer structures induced by albumin. *Chem Phys Lipids,* 2006 144, 137-145.

Lee, SR; Kim, HK; Youm, JB; Dizon, LA; Song, IS; Jeong, SH; Seo, DY; Ko, KS; Rhee, BD; Kim, N; Han, J. Non-genomic effect of glucocorticoids on cardiovascular system. *Pflugers Arch,* 2012 [Epub ahead of print] DOI 10.1007/s00424-012-1155-2.

Li, YH; Yan, ZQ; Brauner, A; Tullus, K. Meconium induces expression of inducible NO synthase and activation of NF-κB in rat alveolar macrophages. *Pediatr Res,* 2001 49, 820-825.

Long, F; Wang, YX; Liu, L; Zhou, J; Cui, RY; Jiang, CL. Rapid nongenomic inhibitory effects of glucocorticoids on phagocytosis and superoxide anion production by macrophages. *Steroids*, 2005 70, 55-61.

Lopez-Rodriguez, E; Echaide, M; Cruz, A; Taeusch, HW; Perez-Gil, J. Meconium impairs pulmonary surfactant by a combined action of cholesterol and bile acids. *Biophys J,* 2011 100, 646-655.

Lösel, R; Wehling, M. Nongenomic actions of steroid hormones. *Nat Rev Mol Cell Biol*, 2003 4, 46-56.

McColl, A; Michlewska, S; Dransfield, I; Rossi, AG. Effects of glucocorticoids on apoptosis and clearance of apoptotic cells. *ScientificWorldJournal*, 2007 7, 1165-1181.

Mokra, D; Calkovska, A; Tonhajzerova, I; Petraskova, M; Bulikova, J; Redfors, B; Javorka, K. Intratracheal budesonide improved the lung functions in meconium-instilled rabbits without side effects on cardiovascular functions. *Eur Respir J*, 2007a 30 Suppl 51, 396p.

Mokra, D; Mokry, J; Drgova, A; Bulikova, J; Petraskova, M; Calkovska, A. Single-dose vs. two-dose dexamethasone effects on lung inflammation and airway reactivity in meconium-instilled rabbits. *J Physiol Pharmacol,* 2007b 58 (Suppl 5), 379-387.

Mokra, D; Mokry, J; Drgova, A; Petraskova, M; Bulikova, J, Calkovska, A. Intratracheally administered corticosteroids improve lung function in meconium-instilled rabbits. *J Physiol Pharmacol,* 2007c 58 (Suppl 5), 389-398.

Mokra, D; Calkovska, A; Tonhajzerova, I; Petraskova, M; Bulikova, J; Redfors, B. Dexamethasone treatment improved lung functions in meconium-instilled rabbits, but influenced cardiovascular variables. *Bratisl Med J,* 2008a 109, 95-101.

Mokra, D; Drgova, A; Mokry, J; Bulikova, J; Pullmann, R; Durdik, P; Petraskova, M; Calkovska, A. Combination of budesonide and aminophylline diminished acute lung injury in animal model of meconium aspiration syndrome. *J Physiol Pharmacol,* 2008b 59 Suppl 6, 461-471.

Mokra, D; Tonhajzerova, I; Mokry, J; Drgova, A; Petraskova, M; Calkovska, A; Javorka, K. Rapid cardiovascular effects of dexamethasone in rabbits with meconium-induced acute lung injury. *Can J Physiol Pharmacol,* 2008c 86, 804-814.

Mokra, D; Mokry, J. Meconium aspiration syndrome. From pathomechanisms to treatment. 1st Edition. New York: Nova Science Publishers; 2010.

Mokry, J; Mokra, D; Antosova, M; Bulikova, J; Calkovska, A; Nosalova, G. Dexamethasone alleviates meconium-induced airway hyperresponsiveness and lung inflammation in rabbits. *Pediatr Pulmonol,* 2006 41, 55-60.

Nimmo, AJ; Carstairs, JR; Patole, SK; Whitehall, J; Davidson, K; Vink, R. Intratracheal administration of glucocorticoids using surfactant as a vehicle. *Clin Exp Pharmacol Physiol,* 2002 29, 661-665.

Ochs, M; Schüttler, M; Stichtenoth, G; Herting, E. Morphological alterations of exogenous surfactant inhibited by meconium can be prevented by dextran. *Respir Res,* 2006 7, 86.

Pallem, V; Kaviratna, AS; Chimote, G; Banerjee, R. Effect of meconium on surface properties of surfactant monolayers and liposomes. *Colloids and Surfaces A: Physicochem Eng Aspects,* 2010 370, 6-14.

Pan, NY; Hui, WS; Tipoe, GL; Taylor, GW; Leung, RY; Lam, WK; Tsang, KW; Mak, JC. Inhibition of pyocyanin-potentiated IL-8 release by steroids in bronchial epithelial cells. *Respir Med,* 2006 100, 1614-1622.

Rizzo, MC; Solé, D. Inhaled corticosteroids in the treatment of respiratory allergy: safety vs. efficacy. *J Pediatr (Rio J),* 2006 82, S198-S205.

Rodríguez-Capote, K; Manzanares, D; Haines, T; Possmayer, F. Reactive oxygen species inactivation of surfactant involves structural and functional alterations to surfactant proteins SP-B and SP-C. *Biophys J,* 2006 90, 2808-2821.

Sáenz, A; López-Sánchez, A; Mojica-Lázaro, J; Martínez-Caro, L; Nin, N; Bagatolli, LA; Casals, C. Fluidizing effects of C-reactive protein on lung surfactant membranes: protective role of surfactant protein A. *FASEB J,* 2010 24, 3662-3673.

Salvia-Roiges, MD; Carbonell-Estrany, X; Figueras-Aloy, J; Rodriguez-Miquelez, JM. Efficacy of three treatment schedules in severe meconium aspiration syndrome. *Acta Paediatr,* 2004 93, 60-65.

Sapolsky, RM; Romero, LM; Munck, AU. How do glucocorticoids influence stress responses? Integrating permissive, suppressive, stimulatory, and preparative actions. *Endocrin Rev,* 2000 21, 55-89.

Schäcke, H; Döcke, WD; Asadullah, K. Mechanisms involved in the side effects of glucocorticoids. *Pharmacology & Therapeutics,* 2002 96, 23-43.

Schrama, AJ; de Beaufort, AJ; Sukul, YR; Jansen, SM; Poorthuis, BJ; Berger, HM. Phospholipase A2 is present in meconium and inhibits the activity of pulmonary surfactant: an in vitro study. *Acta Paediatr,* 2001 90, 412-416.

Soukka, H; Halkola, L; Aho, H; Rautanen, M; Kero, P; Kääpä, P. Methylprednisolone attenuates the pulmonary hypertensive response in porcine meconium aspiration. *Pediatr Res,* 1997 42, 145-150.

Soukka, H; Jalonen, J; Kero, P; Kääpä, P. Endothelin-1, atrial natriuretic peptide and pathophysiology of pulmonary hypertension in porcine meconium aspiration. *Acta Paediatr,* 1998a 87, 424-428.

Soukka, H; Viinika, L; Kääpä, P. Involvement of thromboxane A_2 and prostacyclin in the early pulmonary hypertension after porcine meconium aspiration. *Pediatr Res,* 1998b 44, 838-842.

Soukka, HR; Ahotupa, M; Ruutu, M; Kääpä, PO. Meconium stimulates neutrophil oxidative burst. *Am J Perinatol,* 2002 19, 279-284.

Stellato, C. Post-transcriptional and nongenomic effects of glucocorticoids. *Proc Am Thorac Soc*, 2004 1, 255-263.

Suchomski, SJ; Cummings, JJ. A randomized trial of inhaled versus intravenous steroids in ventilator-dependent preterm infants. *J Perinatol,* 2002 22, 196-203.

Sun, B; Curstedt, T; Robertson, B. Surfactant inhibition in experimental meconium aspiration. *Acta Paediatr,* 1993 82, 182-189.

Sun, HW; Miao, CY; Liu, L; Zhou, J; Su, DF; Wang, YX; Jiang, CL. Rapid inhibitory effect of glucocorticoids on airway smooth muscle contractions in guinea pigs. *Steroids,* 2006 71, 154-159.

Thieringer, R; Le Grand, CB; Carbin, L; Cai, TQ; Wong, B; Wright, SD; Hermanowski-Vosatka, A. 11 Beta-hydroxysteroid dehydrogenase type 1 is induced in human monocytes upon differentiation to macrophages. *J Immunol*, 2001 167, 30-35.

Tomlinson, JW; Walker, EA; Bujalska, I; Draper, N; Lavery, GG; Cooper, MS; Hewison, M; Stewart, PM. 11β-Hydroxysteroid dehydrogenase type 1: a tissue-specific regulator of glucocorticoid response. *Endocr Rev* 2004 25, 831-866.

Tripathi, S; Saili, A; Dutta, R. Inflammatory markers in meconium induced lung injury in neonates and effect of steroids on their levels: a randomized controlled trial. *Indian J Med Microbiol,* 2007 25, 103-107.

Tripathi, S; Saili, A. The effect of steroids on the clinical course and outcome of neonates with meconium aspiration syndrome. *J Trop Pediatr,* 2007 53, 8-12.

Tyler, DC; Murphy, J; Cheney, FW. Mechanical and chemical damage to lung tissue caused by meconium aspiration. *Pediatrics,* 1978 62, 454-459.

Ullian, ME. The role of corticosteroids in the regulation of vascular tone. *Cardiovasc Res,* 1999 41, 55-64.

Vázquez Nava, F; Salas Ramírez, E; Sánchez Núncio, HR; Saldivar González, AH; Beltrán Saldaña, J; Cadena Mata, D; Pérez Rodríguez, P; Pérez Martin, J; Almeida, VM; Guidos Fogelbach, G. Meconium aspiration syndrome, parental atopy and asthma symptoms in children under two years old. *Rev Alerg Mex,* 2006 53, 130-135.

Verriére, VA; Hynes, D; Faherty, S; Devaney, J; Bousquet, J; Harvey, BJ; Urbach, V. Rapid effects of dexamethasone on intracellular pH and Na^+/H^+ exchanger activity in human bronchial epithelial cells. *J Biol Chem,* 2005 280, 35807-35814.

Vidyasagar, D; Zagariya, A. Studies of meconium-induced lung injury: inflammatory cytokine expression and apoptosis. *J Perinatol,* 2008 28, S102-S107.

Walker, BR. Extra-adrenal regeneration of glucocorticoids by 11beta-hydroxysteroid dehydrogenase type 1: physiological regulator and pharmacological target for energy partitioning. *Proc Nutr Soc,* 2007 66, 1-8.

Walker, BR. Glucocorticoids and cardiovascular disease. *Eur J Endocrinol,* 2007 157, 545-559.

Wang, J; Zhang, L; Walther, SM. Administration of aerosolized terbutaline and budesonide reduces chlorine gas-induced acute lung injury. *J Trauma,* 2004 56, 850-862.

Wehling, M. Specific nongenomic actions of steroid hormones. *Ann Rev Physiol,* 1997 59, 365-393.

Whitworth, JA; Mangos, GJ; Kelly, JJ. Cushing, cortisol and cardiovascular disease. *Hypertension*, 2000 36, 912-916.

Wu, JM; Yeh, TF; Wang, JY; Lin, YJ; Hsieh, WS; Lin, CH. The role of pulmonary inflammation in the development of pulmonary hypertension in newborn with meconium aspiration syndrome (MAS). *Pediatr Pulmonol,* 1999 Suppl 18, 205-208.

Yamada, T; Minakami, H; Matsubara, S; Yatsuda, T; Kohmura, Y; Sato, I. Meconium-stained amniotic fluid exhibits chemotactic activity for polymorphonuclear leukocytes in vitro. *J Reprod Immunol,* 2000 46, 21-30.

Yeh, TF; Lin HC; Chang CH; Wu TS; Su BH; Li TC; Pyati S; Tsai CH. Early intratracheal instillation of budesonide using surfactant as a vehicle to prevent chronic lung disease in preterm infants: a pilot study. *Pediatrics,* 2008 121, e1310-e1318.

Yeh, TF; Srinivasan, G; Harris, V; Pildes, RS. Hydrocortisone therapy in meconium aspiration syndrome: a controlled study. *J Pediatr,* 1977 90, 140-143.

Zhou, J; Kang, ZM; Xie, QM; Liu, C; Lou, SJ; Chen, YZ; Jiang, CL. Rapid nongenomic effects of glucocorticoids on allergic asthma reaction in the guinea pig. *J Endocrinol,* 2003 177, R1-R4.

Zuo, YY; Veldhuize, RA; Neumann, AW; Petersen, NO; Possmayer, F. Current perspectives in pulmonary surfactant - Inhibition, enhancement and evaluation. *Biochim Biophys Acta,* 2008 1778, 1947-1977.

Reviewed by:

Jana Plevkova, MD., PhD., Assoc. Prof., Department of Pathological Physiology, Jessenius Faculty of Medicine, Comenius University, Martin, Slovakia;

Martin Wawruch, MD., PhD., Assoc. Prof., Department of Pharmacology and Clinical Pharmacology, Faculty of Medicine, Comenius University, Bratislava, Slovakia.

In: Neonatal Care: New Research
Editors: F. Koubek and J. Linser

ISBN: 978-1-62618-454-1

Chapter 4

HYPERBILIRUBINEMIA, AUDITORY NEUROPATHY AND PRELINGUALLY DEAFNESS: EVIDENCE LINKING

Francesco Martines[1,*] and Pietro Salvago[2]

[1]Università degli Studi di Palermo, Dipartimento di Biomedicina Sperimentale e Neuroscienze Cliniche,
Sezione di Otorinolaringoiatria, Palermo, Italy
[2]Università degli Studi di Palermo, Dipartimento di Biotecnologie Mediche e Medicina Forenze, Sezione di Audiologia, Palermo, Italy

ABSTRACT

Among risk factors for sensorineural hearing loss (SNHL), hyperbilirubinemia, a clinical-laboratoristic condition characterized by an excess of bilirubin in the blood, can play an important role in the development of deafness. Newborns are particularly susceptible to suffer from this pathology because of the great amount of bilirubin produced from the red cell turnover combined with the immaturity of enzymatic systems involved in bilirubin excretion.

Research suggested that the pathogenetic mechanism responsible of the hearing impairment consists in the deposition of bilirubin in the

* Correspondence to: Francesco Martines, PhD. Via Autonomia Siciliana 70- 90143 Palermo (Italy). Tel.: 0039-091.545666; Fax: 0039-091.6554271. E-mail: francesco.martines@ unipa.it; E-mail: francescomartines@ hotmail.com.

cochlear nuclei and in the auditory pathways. This condition occurs more frequently when total serum bilirubin exceeds 20-25 mg/dl and the unconjugated bilirubin in excess can overcome the Blood-Brain-Barrier (BBB) performing a neurotoxic action.

The main causes of hyperbilirubinemia are Rh and ABO maternal-fetal incompatibility, red cells' morphologic (as spherocytosis and elliptocytosis) and enzymatic (Glucose-6-phosphate dehydrogenase deficiency, Crigler-Najjar' syndrome, Gilbert' syndrome) defects.

Literature data is full of studies that investigate the role of hyperbilirubinemia in the development of SNHL trying to establish a total serum bilirubin (TSB) cut-off above whom newborns can be considered at high SNHL risk; nevertheless, a clear bilirubin threshold has not been defined yet. Surely, as recommended by the Joint Committee on infant hearing (JCIH) in its Position Statement of 2007, all jaundiced newborns requiring exchange transfusion should be assessed to early identify the presence of an hearing impairment.

Recent studies conducted through audiometry, otoacoustic emissions (OAEs) and auditory brainstem response (ABR), reported, in patients who suffered from hyperbilirubinemia, the presence of a cochlear and retrochlear, mainly bilateral, hearing loss with an audiometric pattern characterized by an involvement of the high frequencies.

Furthermore, among SNHL newborns who suffered from hyperbilirubinemia, it is more probable to observe a particular audiologic disease called "auditory neuropathy spectrum disorder" (ANSD), often misunderstood because of its characteristic audiologic profile (present OAEs, not recordable ABR, absence of the acoustic reflexes) that results from a damage of the cochlear inner hair cells, their synapses with the cochlear nerve or the cochlear nerve itself but with the preservation of the outer hair cells.

Introduction

Occurring in about 60% of newborns, hyperbilirubinemia is a pathologic condition involving neonates when the amount of bilirubin in the blood exceeds 5 mg/dl, causing the yellowish pigmentation of the skin, the sclerae and other mucous membranes (neonatal jaundice). Additionally, high levels of serum bilirubin are responsible of neuronal injury and severe clinical consequences as hearing loss and kernicterus.

Hearing involvement regards mainly auditory pathway, with the deposition of free bilirubin in brainstem sites as cochlear nuclei, the superior olivary complex, the lateral lemnisci, the trapezoid bodies and the inferior colliculi of the midbrain. The localization of damage in the auditory nervous system corresponds to a particular hearing disease, known as "auditory neuropathy spectrum disorder" (ANSD), whose audiological features are the presence of otoacustic emissions (OAEs) and/or cochlear microponics (CM), recordable auditory brainstem responses (ABR) and absent stapedial reflexes. Clinically ANSD children show a behavioural audiometry with variable pattern of hearing loss that not correlate with their main hearing problem: the extreme difficulty understanding speech especially in presence of environmental noise.

Even if a bilirubin threshold that places infants at certain risk of hearing impairment has not been defined yet, it was proposed by Joint Committee on infant hearing (JCIH) in its Position Statement of 2007 to undergo all jaundiced newborns requiring exchange transfusion to hearing screening programs. Furthermore, considering the frequent association between severe hyperbilirubinemia (bilirubin levels >20 mg/dl) and ANSD, neonates presenting this risk factor should be assessed at the time of first evaluation with the contemporary recording of OAEs and ABR to make an early diagnosis.

Bilirubin Metabolism and Main Causes of Neonatal Jaundice

Bilirubin is a tetrapyrrole produced from the catabolism of hemoglobin, myoglobin and other cells' components like cytochromes; it derives approximately 75% from hemolytic processes and about 25% from ineffective erythropoiesis. Bilirubin metabolism begins with the conversion of hemoglobin to biliverdin by heme oxygenase and continues with the transformation of biliverdin, in a reaction catalyzed by biliverdin reductase, to unconjugated (or indirect) bilirubin (about the 80% of total blood bilirubin). This form of bilirubin (nonpolar and lipid soluble) is bound to serum albumin and sent to the liver. Here bilirubin is bound to one or two molecules of glucuronic acid forming the so-called conjugated (or direct) bilirubin. This is a water-soluble, nontoxic glucuronide that results from the action of an enzyme called diphosphate-glucuronyltransferase (UDPGT), that catalyzes, in the hepatocytes, the binding process of bilirubin to glucuronic acid before bilirubin's excretion in the biliary system. Conjugated bilirubin is eliminated in stool, but also broken down by bowel flora to unconjugated bilirubin, which is then adsorbed by the intestinal mucosa and returns to the liver via the portal vein (enterohepatic circulation).

All pathologic processes that interfere with bilirubin metabolism can cause an increase (from mild to severe) of blood bilirubin concentration and so an overcome of its physiological levels: this condition is called "hyperbilirubinemia" and its first clinical sign is jaundice, a yellowish discoloration of the skin and the conjunctival membranes over the sclerae.

In newborns, differently from adults, jaundice appears when total serum bilirubin (TSB) exceeds 5 mg/dl; it is clinically assessed by quickly pressing and releasing the skin. This exam, called "blanching", causes the skin to become pale, so it is possible to see if the skin is yellowed as blood returns to the blanched area.

Several diseases are responsible of neonatal hyperbilirubinemia, but the more common is represented by physiologic jaundice that occurs around 60% of newborns during their first week of life (with a peak of 80% in pre-term babies). This kind of jaundice appears generally between 24-72 hours of age with a maximum intensity seen on 4-5th day in term and 7th day in preterm neonates. Normally it does not exceed 15 mg/dl of total bilirubin and it is due to an increased breakdown of red blood cells (RBC) and to the immaturity of the hepatocytes enzymatic systems (resulting in a defective conjugation and a decreased excretion of bilirubin).

Concerning jaundice etiology, it is possible to classify the main causes of hyperbilirubinemia in two different groups depending on the prevalent form of bilirubin accumulated in the blood (indirect or direct).

The main conditions causing high blood level of unconjugated bilirubin are: first, increased lysis of RBCs due to isoimmunization (blood group incompatibility: Rh, ABO and minor blood groups), RBC enzyme defects (Glucose-6-phosphate dehydrogenase deficiency, pyruvate kinase deficiency), RBC structural abnormalities (hereditary spherocytosis, elliptocytosis), infection and sequestered blood (cephalohematoma, bruising, intracranial hemorrhage); second, decreased hepatic uptake and conjugation of bilirubin due to Gilbert Syndrome, Crigler Najjar Syndrome, pyloric stenosis and hypothyroidism.

The Rh maternal-fetal incompatibility is the major cause of jaundice with a large amount of indirect bilirubin produced by an increased destruction of RBC. This hemolytic process occurs in some second or subsequent pregnancies of Rh negative women where the fetus is Rh positive; during pregnancy, RBC from the fetus can get into the mother's bloodstream and so mother's immune system treats the Rh-positive fetal cells as if they were a foreign substance and makes antibodies against them. Newborns do not appear jaundiced at birth, but severe anemia can lead to hydrops and death. After birth, infants may develop hyperbilirubinemia rapidly.

ABO incompatibility is a hemolytic disease caused by a reaction of maternal anti-A or anti-B antibodies with fetal A or B antigens. It is almost exclusively in type O mothers and generally with a hemolytic anemia of mild degree and a 24-72 hours of age onset.

A great increase of indirect bilirubin in the bloodstream can be observed in newborns with two autosomal dominant genetic diseases, hereditary elliptocytosis and spherocytosis. The RBC of these infants are more susceptible to be destroyed by spleen because of their cytoskeletal anomalies determined by mutations of proteins like spectrin or ankyrin. With an incidence of 1:4000 babies, hereditary elliptocytosis is a RBC disorder whose clinical expression (hemolysis and hyperbilirubinemia) is unusual in the newborn period. Neonates with hereditary spherocitosis instead, present in the 50% of cases hemolytic anemia, hyperbilirubinemia, reticulocytosis and increased erythrocyte osmotic fragility.

Other important genetic causes of neonatal jaundice are glucose-6-phosphate dehydrogenase (G6PD) deficiency, Crigler-Najjar' syndrome and Gilbert' syndrome. The first one is an X-linked disease in which RBC are unable to activate the pentose phosphate metabolic pathway and consequently cannot defend against oxidative stress. G6PD deficiency affects almost exclusively male subjects in which the hemolytic process is triggered by infections, severe stress, certain foods and drugs. The presentation is heterogeneous and hyperbilirubinemia occurs between 24-72 hours of life.

Crigler-Najjar' syndrome and Gilbert' syndrome instead are characterized by mutation of an enzyme involved in bilirubin's metabolism and called "glucuronosyltransferase", whose reduced function or severe deficiency can lead to different clinical manifestations, from mild jaundice to an extremely serious brain dysfunction known as "Kernicterus".

From 1 to 10 breastfed infants present in the first week of life the "breastfeeding jaundice". The cause is thought to be inadequate milk intake, leading to dehydration, low caloric intake and also delayed passage of meconium with consequent increased enterohepatic reuptake of bilirubin leading to hyperbilirubinemia.

Breast milk jaundice is far less common and occurs in about 1 in 200 newborns. The jaundice occurs after the first week of life, but it often reaches its peak during the second or third week. Breast milk jaundice can be caused by unidentified components of mother's milk that decrease the infant's liver's ability to break down bilirubin.

Finally neonatal hyperbilirubinemia can be caused by hepatocellular damage or reduced biliary excretion with consequent high plasma levels of direct bilirubin. These pathogenetic mechanisms determine a jaundice (defined as "cholestatic") in newborns who suffer from idiopathic neonatal hepatitis, intrahepatic or extrahepatic biliary atresia, total parenteral nutrition, perinatal asphyxia and metabolic disorders (e.g. Alpha-1 antitrypsin deficiency, Glycogen storage disorders).

From the Neurotoxic Effects to the Auditory Pathway Damage

Although the molecular pathogenesis of neuronal cell injury by bilirubin is not completely understood, it is demonstrated that the damage starts involving cell membrane and leads to an excessive release and impaired reuptake of glutamate, to mitochondrial energy failure and increased intracellular calcium concentration (with the activation of apoptotic pathways).

The risk of neuronal injury by bilirubin is primarily determined by the blood concentration of unconjugated bilirubin and hydrogen ion (pH). Unconjugated bilirubin, when unbound to albumin or in presence of displacing drugs (such as sulphonamides), can cross freely the Blood-Brain Barrier (BBB) reaching interstitial and cerebrospinal fluid. Moreover, pathologic conditions like sepsis, acidosis and hypoxia may decrease the bilirubin binding affinity of albumin. Bilirubin bound to albumin does not enter the brain except when the BBB is disrupted.

Literature data is full of studies that tried to understand which level of bilirubin could be considered "safe", but actually a sure bilirubin threshold is not defined. A condition of severe hyperbilirubinemia, at high risk for neurologic and audiologic disorders, occurs when TSB value overcomes 20 mg/dl or increase of > 0.20 mg/dL/hr. However, disturbances of the hearing function have already been found at lower values. In fact, in case of bilirubin levels of less than 20 mg/dl, auditory brainstem responses (ABR) often showed prolonged latencies, which proved to be reversible [1, 2, 3, 4]. In contrast, in 50% of the affected children non-reversible changes (significantly elevated latencies or no responses up to maximum sound pressure levels) were found after diagnosing TSB-level over 20 mg/dl [1, 5, 6]. Furthermore, lower

TSB level could be responsible of neurological consequences in premature and very low birth weight (VLBW) newborns due to their susceptibility to suffer from hypoxia, acidosis and sepsis.

The BBB plays a role in protection of the nervous tissues from bilirubin toxic action and its disruption produces diffuse yellow staining but not the specific pattern of kernicterus [7].

Different studies suggested the presence of an ATP dependent transporter molecules whose function is to export unconjugated bilirubin; the main objective of this physiologic mechanism is to remove bilirubin from the brain and maintain the concentration gradient of bilirubin from plasma to cerebrospinal fluid (CSF) [8, 9, 10].

Bilirubin brain toxicity is correlated with neuronal susceptibility. In fact, investigations conducted by Shapiro (2003) revealed the existence of a critical period during which elevated levels of bilirubin in blood could seriously obstacle nervous tissue development.

This theory was hypnotized examining cerebella of jaundiced Gunn rats made toxic at various developmental ages; it was evidenced a relationship between time of exposure and susceptibility to bilirubin: neurons undergoing differentiation were the most susceptible to cell death, while those that were slightly more or less mature showed only transient changes or seemed to be much less sensitive [10].

It was also suggested that bilirubin can interfere with intracellular calcium homeostasis by altering function and expression of calcium/calmodulin kinase II, by selectively decreasing calcium binding proteins in susceptible brainstem areas and increasing intracellular calcium in cultured neurons and by sensitizing the cell to other injuries or triggering apoptosis. Another way to kill cells is performing a neuronal excitotoxic action through an excessive release and impaired reuptake of glutamate, the primary excitatory neurotransmitter in the Central Nervous System (CNS) with resultant over activation of excitatory amino acid receptors. Finally, it can inhibit mitochondrial respiration and energy production [11, 12, 13, 14].

Bilirubin induces ultra structural changes acting directly on mitochondrial membranes and disrupting lipid polarity, fluidity and protein order. It leads to increased membrane permeability [15], mitochondrial depolarization [16], collapse of mitochondrial transmembrane potential, release of cytochrome-c and activation of the intrinsic apoptotic pathway.

Overall, the main factors influencing different patterns of damage and consequently the clinical expression are the amount and duration of exposure to free bilirubin, the susceptibility of the developing nervous tissue, the relative amount of necrosis or apoptosis process occurred and the surviving neurons' functionality and sensitivity to other stress factors.

Bilirubin neurotoxic action has different targets, particularly basal ganglia of the brain and auditory nervous system, with a variable clinical expression, from isolated hearing impairment to kernicterus, a severe neurologic disease. Kernicterus results from a selective damage to the globus pallidus, substantia nigra reticulata, subthalamic nucleus (STN), brainstem auditory, vestibular and oculomotor nuclei, hippocampus and cerebellum [17].

The classic clinical manifestation is a tetrad, which includes deafness or dysfunction of the auditory system, movement disorders (such as athetosis, dystonia and hypotonia), oculomotor disturbances (especially paresis or upgaze) and dental enamel hypoplasia of the deciduous teeth.

Shapiro and Nakamura investigated the localization of damage in the auditory system through an immunohistochemistry analysis of the expression of two calcium binding proteins (calbindin and parvalbumin) in brains of jaundiced Gunn rats; the main neuroanatomical sites targeted by bilirubin damage resulted cochlear nuclei, the superior olivary complex, the lateral lemnisci, the trapezoid bodies and the inferior colliculi of the midbrain. The cell bodies of the auditory nerve in the spiral ganglia of the cochlea appeared abnormal (reduced cell size and density) with a selective loss of large myelinated fibers in the auditory nerve, whereas the smaller fibers were normal or less affected.

Finally inner ear, thalamus and cortical auditory pathways were not involved in damage, even in those Gunn rats who presented severely abnormal or absent auditory brainstem responses.[18]

The auditory nervous system abnormalities previously exposed, either alone or in combination with sensory loss, are suggested by reports of decreased binaural fusion, auditory aphasia and poor speech perception, particularly in subjects with audiometric tests that indicate normal thresholds [19, 20, 21, 22, 23].

In fact, the auditory damage from hyperbilirubinemia differs from the more frequent classic "sensorineural" hearing loss (SNHL) and is associated with a dysfunction at the level of the auditory brainstem or nerve. This auditory dysfunction causes a condition currently known as Auditory Neuropathy Spectrum Disorder (ANSD), which is functionally defined as absent or abnormal ABR with evidence of normal inner ear function assessed by either OAE or cochlear microphonic (CM) responses.

Audiological Features: Hearing Loss and Auditory Neuropathy Spectrum Disorder (ANSD)

Different studies reported the prevalence of hyperbilirubinemia among SNHL infants with variable results depending on the characteristics of the cohorts examined and on the distribution of other risk factors less or more associated with auditory dysfunction and hearing impairment [24, 25, 26, 27, 28].

Hyperbilirubinemia (specifically TSB level that requires an exchange transfusion) is considered from JCIH a risk factor for development of SNHL, with researches evidencing audiometric pattern with a predominantly high-frequency bilateral and symmetric hearing loss with recruitment and abnormal loudness growth functions [20, 21, 22] that correlates with pathologic lesions in the cochlear nuclei [29, 30].

Combining measures of ABR, CM responses and/or OAE the sites of altered functions can be identified as affecting one or more of the components comprising the auditory periphery including outer hair cells, auditory nerve and auditory brain structures.

ABR is a series of electrical potentials generated in response to activation of auditory pathway structures. It is the expression of neural activity in the auditory nerve, the cochlear nucleus in the pons, and fiber tracts of midbrain lateral lemniscus leading into the inferior colliculus (waves I-V). A parameter evaluated is latency of each wave, a time interval in milliseconds from stimulus onset to peak of each wave. Transient auditory dysfunction represents the early acute and reversible ABR changes secondary to moderate hyperbilirubinemia instead of SNHL that represents the chronic and irreversible consequence of severe or prolonged hyperbilirubinemia.

Wennberg (1982) and Kurivama (1986) described changes in ABR before and after exchange transfusion in term neonates with hyperbilirubinemia [31, 32]. These bilirubin-induced ABR changes progress from reversible prolongation of the absolute wave latencies followed by reduced wave amplitude and ultimately the impossibility to recognize an identifiable wave [31, 32, 33]. The waves reappeared and latencies decreased following exchange blood transfusion; so ABR improves as the bilirubin level falls suggesting that ABR can be a useful instrument to investigate bilirubin-induced neurotoxicity in term infants [31, 32].

Different studies have demonstrated a relationship between ABR changes and bilirubin damage involving auditory nerve and/or brainstem. Kaga et al.

assessing 25 children affected by kernicterus at 1 to 5 years of age evidenced the presence of ABR anomalies (absence of ABR or wave I abnormalities without increase in interpeak intervals) suggesting lesions in the auditory nerve [34].

A second tool helpful to evaluate cochlear function are CM, receptor potentials generated by both inner and outer cochlear hair cells. Since the dominant type of hair cell is outer, one would expect that the amplitude of CM derives predominantly from outer rather than inner hair cells, that can also be identified in the ABR by separately averaging potentials to condensation and rarefaction stimuli to define phafe reversed components in the two averages. If the condensation and rarefaction stimuli are presented in the altering fashion, the CM to each polarity stimulus cancel and do not appear in the ABR average. In hyperbilirubinemic newborns, despite an absence of ABR waves, CM response persists and may even be excessively large, the so called 'giant' CM responses.

Chisin evidenced the preservation of cochlear microphonic (CM) and absent or abnormal ABR responses in 13 SNHL jaundiced infants greater than 32 weeks gestational age [35]. Furthermore, he observed a difference in prevalence of SNHL and cerebral palsy between infants with peak TSB levels < 20 mg/dL and those with peak TSB levels > 20 mg/dL, suggesting that auditory toxicity occurs at a lower level of hyperbilirubinemia than cerebral palsy due to a particular susceptibility to bilirubin injury by auditory nervous pathway [36]

OAEs are weak sounds generated by motile elements in the cochlear outer hair cells and can be detected in response to sound stimulation by a small microphone placed in the external ear canal. If cochlear outer hair cells are damaged, OAEs can't be recorded. As observed by Nickisch in his 5-years follow-up of 15 infants who suffered from hyperbilirubinemia, OAEs were dectected in 7 children in presence of an abnormal ABR (ANSD), whereas in the others OAEs were absent. Furthermore, two cases presented OAEs initially measurable, later extincted [37].

Generally deaf children present SNHL with a 0.5-15% of them affected by a ANSD [38]. As showed in table 1, a history of hyperbilirubinemia can be found in about 50% of ANSD children [24, 38, 39, 40, 41]. Main etiologies are also perinatal hypoxia, prematurity and genetic causes (mainly mutations of OTOF gene, encoding for a protein called "Otoferlin" which control neurotrasmettitori release by cochlear inner hair cells. Research suggested that ANSD is due to an abnormality or lesion at one of these points: the level of the cochlear inner hair cells, the synapse between the inner hair cells and auditory nerve or at the auditory nerve itself [42]. It has been proposed that the firing in the nerve is desynchronised in its transmission along the neural pathway. Children who suffer from ANSD present an hearing loss of variable degree, from mild to profound, with extremely poor speech discrimination regardless of degree of hearing impairment. This inconsistency between speech discrimination and degree of hearing is the first suggestion that a deaf patient may have ANSD. In order to confirm a diagnosis of ANSD, the following three characteristics should be evident: extreme difficulty "hearing" in various situations regardless of hearing level, absent or abnormal auditory neural function and normal cochlear function. So the following audiologic test should be performed to recognize ANSD profile: recording of ABR, study of stapedial reflexes, air and bone conduction audiometry, evaluation of OAEs and speech discrimination testing.

Table 1. Published studies reporting ANSD associated to hyperbilirubinemia among SNHL Infants cohorts

Author	Year	N° of Infants	Age range	Audiological assessment	ANSD group	
					N° (%)	N° of children suffering from hyperbilirubinemia (%)*
Bielecki et al.	2012	352	0-1 Month	OAEs ABR Impedenzometry	18 (5.11%)	7 (38.9%)
Martines et al.	2012	47	4-20 Weeks	OAEs ABR Impedenzometry	4 (8.51%)	2 (50%)
Hossam Sanyelbhaa Talaat et al.	2009	112	6-32 Months	CMs ABR Behavioral audiometry	15 (13.3%)	6 (40%)
Madden et al.	2002	428	1-60 Months	OAEs ABR Behavioral audiometry	22 (5.14%)	11 (50%)
Berg et al.	2005	477	0-22 Months	OAEs ABR	115 (24.1%)	51 (44.3%)

* The percentage is related to the cases of ANSD.

ANSD is characterized by an absent or poorly defined ABR with preserved OAE and/or preserved CM responses [43, 44, 45]. In most cases of ANSD, ABRs performed at 80 db are usually limited to early/fast waves (CM) that exhibit fixed-latency function and complete phase reversal between rarefaction and condensation stimuli [46]. In some instances of ANSD, the ABR may show a wave V, but with decreased amplitude and increased latency [43, 47]. ANSD children present a behavioral audiometry that can vary greatly anywhere from normal hearing to severe hearing loss showing unusual audiometric pattern. Stapedial reflexes are generally absent. Clinically these patients also experience great difficulty in understanding speech, particularly in the presence of background noise.

Considering the ANSD audiological features, it is recommended to evaluate newborns who suffered from hyperbilirubinemia (especially those whose bilirubin levels exceed 20 mg/dl) with a complete audiologic assessment to reduce the risk to overlook ANSD. In fact, OAE testing (commonly used as firs step screening tool) is quick and easy to do; however, abnormalities of the afferent inner hair cells, the auditory nerve, or auditory brainstem pathways do not alter the OAEs. ABR instead, would detect all children with a significant clinical hearing loss independently from their audiologic profile allowing to an early intervention.

Prelingually Deafness in Jaundiced Newborns: Speech Perception, Early Diagnosis and Rehabilitation

It is well recognized that hearing is necessary to reach a correct speech and language development, making possible an adequate communication and learning. Specifically, when hearing loss occurs in the first years of life, all this goals can't be achieved without an early diagnosis and an appropriate rehabilitation. In fact, if deafness is overlooked or misunderstood, it can determine dramatic consequences on the child's quality of life interesting different levels of his psychological and social growth: first, hearing impairment causes delay in the development of receptive and expressive communication skills (vocabulary, sentence structure and speaking are compromised); particularly ANSD children present with difficulty understanding speech that is not correlated with the audiometric threshold.

Second, deaf children have difficulty with all areas of academic achievement (especially reading and mathematical concepts) with lower capacity of concentration and decreased attention at school. The result is a gap in learning that increases as they progress through school between them and their normal hearings peers.

Finally, hearing impaired children often report feeling isolated, without friends and unhappy in school; in fact their hearing deficit influences negatively their socialization, their interaction with other children and their emotional development with a compromised personal and relational growth.

So, considering the severe effects of hearing loss on child development, a diagnosis made until the 6th month of life is necessary to counteract the progressively irreversible damage determined by auditory deprivation. This objective can be achieved by hearing screening programs, remembering that, for all late preterm and term infants with severe hyperbilirubinemia (TSB > 20 mg/dl) or TSB level at which exchange transfusion is required, a screening with OAEs must be considered insufficient instead of a complete audiologic evaluation that should reduce consistently the risk of unidentified ANSD infants.

Once deafness is diagnosed, the kind and degree of hearing impairment influences the intervention choice, whose only purpose is to provide access to language and child's environment in most efficacious manner.

ANSD infants have a more complex rehabilitation process than the classic SNHL peers due to ANSD audiological features. In fact the choice of intervention is more difficult because of the not clear knowledge of the pathophysiology of ANSD jointed with the variability of the auditory damage location. A trial with hearing aids is essential but in ANSD children ABR, that normally provides hearing threshold information, is generally absent or abnormal at high levels; so we must have behavioral threshold data prior to fitting hearing aids, that means waiting until 6-12 months of life (or later) before this data is reliably available. Monitoring of speech and language development as well as auditory skills should be undertaken to help assess the impact of amplification. According to Rance, only the 50% of ANSD infants could show benefit from hearing aids [48]. The remaining 50% represents a potential candidate to cochlear implant intervention.

Cochlear implantation is actually the management option of choice for ANSD children with audiograms in the severe/profound range or significant auditory processing difficulties. Most reported cases have shown normal device function and post-implant speech perception performance broadly similar with their implanted SNHL peers [38, 49, 50]

The ways in which perception is improved by the cochlear implant in ears with ANSD is currently not completely understood. After implantation, most of the ANSD children present recordable brainstem potentials to electrical stimulation, where previously to acoustic stimulation they had not.

Probably it is explainable hypothesizing an increase in the number of neural elements contributing to the ABR (perhaps as a result of by-passing a peripheral abnormality when stimulating the spiral ganglion directly) or an improvement in the synchrony of neural firing in the auditory pathway (perhaps reflecting the fact that the electrical stimuli are presented as a series of discrete pulses rather than analog signals).

However, cochlear implantation could be uneffective due to the presence of an absent or hypoplasic VIIIth nerve; so, before considering cochlear implant surgery, it's necessary to rule out a VIIIth nerve deficiency through Magnetic Resonance Imaging (MRI). Finally, infants with bilaterally absent cochlear nerves are clearly not candidates for amplification or cochlear implantation. In these children it is strongly encouraged the introduction of alternative forms of communication [51].

CONCLUSION

Among prelingually deafness etiologies, neonatal hyperbilirubinemia represents a potential cause of SNHL, with greater probability to suffer from hearing loss in presence of high levels of bilirubin in the blood and also other perinatal risk factors (hypoxia, infections, ototoxic drugs...) that can make CNS more susceptible to bilirubin injury.

Frequently a hearing impairment associated with neonatal hyperbilirubinemia appears as ANSD and represents, differently from the classic kind of SNHL, a challenge for its variable rehabilitative outcomes. In fact the different neuroanatomical sites against which bilirubin performs a neurotoxic action are the main factors influencing the success of rehabilitative intervention. While generally deaf children treated before the age of 2 years, comparing to a normal hearing control group, show normative levels of speech perception performance just at three months post hearing aids/implantation, the ANSD children often does not benefit by trying hearing aids and so cochlear implantation should be considered remembering that, a VIIIth nerve deficiency could make this surgery partially or totally ineffective.

Therefore it's important to underline that the first objective is to prevent hearing loss due to hyperbilirubinemia monitoring newborns till the time of their hospital discharge and treat neonatal jaundice as recommended by the American Academy of Pediatrics [52].

Children suffering from hyperbilirubinemia that requires exchange transfusion should perform a complete audiologic assessment with OAEs and ABR to test cochlear and auditory pathway function and early recognize hearing impairment independently from its audiological characteristics.

REFERENCES

[1] Gupta A.K., Mann S.B.S. (1998). Is auditory brainstem response a bilirubin neurotoxicity marker? *Am J Otolaryngol,* 19, 232–236.

[2] Pallotta R., Minervino M., Sabatino G., Nardini P., Elicio M.R. (1984). Long-term effects of neonatal medium-degree hyperbilirubinemia on brainstem evoked potentials. *Pediatr Med Chir,* 6, 273–276.

[3] Tan K.L., Skurr B.A., Yip Y.Y. (1992). Phototherapy and the brainstem auditory evoked response in neonatal hyperbilirubinemia. *J Pediatr*, 120, 306–308.

[4] Thoma J., Gerull G., Mrowinski D. (1986). A long term study of hearing in children following neonatal hyperbilirubinemia. *Arch Otorhinolaryngol*, 243, 133–137.

[5] Madden C., Rutter M., Hilbert L., Greinwald J., Choo D. (2002). Clinical and audiological features in auditory neuropathy. *Arch Otolaryngol*, 128, 1026–1030.

[6] Shapiro S.M., Rosen J.R., Dixon K.T. (2002). Auditory brainstem responses and auditory neuropathy abnormalities in children with neonatal hyperbilirubinemia who subsequently develop kernicterus. *Pediatr Res,* 51(Part 2), 340A.

[7] Ahlfors C.E. (2001). Bilirubin-albumin binding and free bilirubin. *J Perinatol,* 21 (Suppl 1), S40-S42.

[8] Hansen T.W. (2002). Mechanisms of bilirubin toxicity: clinical implications. *Clin Perinatol,* 29(4), 765-778.

[9] Watchko J.F., Daood M.J., Biniwale M. (2002). Understanding neonatal hyperbilirubinemia in the era of genomics. *Semin Neonatol,* 7(2), 143-152.

[10] Shapiro S.M. (2003). Bilirubin toxicity in the developing nervous system. *Pediatr Neurol*, 29(5), 410-421.

[11] Hansen T.W., Sagvolden T., Bratlid D. (1987). Open-field behavior of rats previously subjected to short-term hyperbilirubinemia with or without blood-brain barrier manipulations. *Brain Res,* 424(1), 26-36.
[12] Hanko E., Hansen T.W., Almaas R., Lindstad J., Rootwelt T. (2005). Bilirubin induces apoptosis and necrosis in human NT2-N neurons. *Pediatr Res,* 57(2), 179-184.
[13] Brito M.A., Brites D., Butterfield D.A. (2004). A link between hyperbilirubinemia, oxidative stress and injury to neocortical synaptosomes. *Brain Res,* 1026(1), 33-43.
[14] Shapiro S.M. (2002). Somatosensory and brainstem auditory evoked potentials in the Gunn rat model of acute bilirubin neurotoxicity. *Pediatr Res,* 52(6), 844-849.
[15] Rodrigues C. M. P., Sola S., Castro R. E., Laires P. A.,Brites D., and Moura J. J. G. (2002b). Perturbation of membrane dynamics in nerve cells as an early event during bilirubin-induced apoptosis. *J Lipid Res,* 43, 885–894.
[16] Keshavan P., Schwemberger S. J., Smith D. L. H., Babcock G. F., and Zucker S. D. (2004). Unconjugated bilirubin induces apoptosis in colon cancer cells by triggering mitochondrial depolarization. *Int J Cancer,* 112, 433–445.
[17] Shapiro S.M. (2010). Chronic bilirubin encephalopathy: diagnosis and outcome. *Semin Fetal Neonatal Med,* 15(3), 157-163.
[18] Shapiro S.M., Nakamura H. (2001). Bilirubin and the auditory system. *J Perinatol,* 21 Suppl 1, S52-55.
[19] Byers R.K., Paine R.S., Crothers B. (1955). Extrapyramidal cerebral palsy with hearing loss following erythroblastosis. *Pediatrics,* 15, 248-254.
[20] Perlstein M.A. (1960). The late clinical syndrome of posticteric encephalopathy. *Pediatr Clin North Am,* 7, 665-687.
[21] Matkin N.D., Carhart R. (1966). Auditory profiles associated with Rh incompatibility. *Arch Otolaryngol,* 84, 502-513.
[22] Ruben R., Lieberman A., Bordley J. (1962). Some observations on cochlear potentials and nerve action potentials in children. *Laryngoscope,* 72, 545-553.
[23] Hardy W.G. (1961). Auditory deficits of the kernicterus child. In: Swinyard CA, ed. *Kernicterus and its importance in cerebral palsy.* Springfield, IL: Charles C. Thomas, 21-228.
[24] Martines F., Salvago P., Bentivegna D., Bartolone A., Dispenza F., Martines E. (2012). Audiologic profile of infants at risk: experience of a

Western Sicily tertiary care centre. *Int J Pediatr Otorhinolaryngol,* 76(9), 1285-1291.

[25] Declau F., Boudewyns A., Van den Ende J., Peeters A., van den Heyning P. (2008). Etiologic and audiologic evaluations after universal neonatal hearing screening: analysis of 170 referred neonates. *Pediatrics,* 121(6), 1119-1126.

[26] Coenraad S., Goedegebure A., van Goudoever J.B., Hoeve L.J. (2010). Risk factors for sensorineural hearing loss in NICU infants compared to normal hearing NICU controls. *Int J Pediatr Otorhinolaryngol,* 74(9), 999-1002.

[27] Sutton G.J., Rowe S.J. (1997). Risk factors for childhood sensorineural hearing loss in the Oxford region. *Br J Audiol,* 31, 39-54.

[28] Mäki-Torkko E.M., Lindholm P.K., Väyrynen M.R., Leisti J.T., Sorri M.J. (1998). Epidemiology of moderate to profound childhood hearing impairments in northern Finland. Any changes in ten years?. *Scand Audiol,* 27(2), 95-103.

[29] Dublin W. (1951). Neurological lesions in erythroblastosis fetalis in relation to nuclear deafness. *Am J Clin Path,* 21, 935-939.

[30] Dublin W. (1986). Central auditory pathology. *Otolaryngol Head Neck Surg,* 95, 363-424.

[31] Wennberg R.P., Ahlfors C.E., Bickers R., McMurtry C.A., Shetter J.L. (1982). Abnormal auditory brainstem response in a newborn infant with hyperbilirubnemia: Improvement with exchange transfusion. *J Pediatr,* 100, 624-626.

[32] Kurivama H., Tomiwa K., Konishi Y., Mikawa H. (1986). Improvement in auditory brainstem response of hyperbilirubinemic infants after exchange transfusion. *Pediatr Neurol,* 2, 127-132.

[33] Amin S.B., Orlando M.S., Merle K.S., Dalzell L.E., Guillet R. (1997). Sequential changes in BAER and their relation to bilirubin levels in neonates less than 32 weeks gestational age. *Pediatr Res,* 41, 135A.

[34] Kaga K., Kitazumi E., Kodama K. (1979). Auditory brainstem responses of kernicterus infants. *Int J Pediatr Otorhinolaryngol,* 1, 255-264.

[35] Chisin R., Perlman N., Sohmer H. (1979). Cochlear and brainstem responses in hearing loss following neonatal hyperbilirubinemia. *Ann Otol Rhinol Laryngol,* 89, 352-357.

[36] Amin S.B. (2004). Clinical assessment of bilirubin-induced neurotoxicity in premature infants. *Semin Perinatol,* 28(5), 340-347.

[37] Nickisch A., Massinger C., Ertl-Wagner B., von Voss H. (2009). Pedaudiologic findings after severe neonatal hyperbilirubinemia. *Eur Arch Otorhinolaryngol,* 266(2), 207-212.
[38] Madden C., Rutter M., Hilbert L., Greinwald J.H., Choo D.I. (2002). Clinical and audiological features in auditory neuropathy. *Arch Otolaryngol Head Neck Surg,* 128(9), 1026-30.
[39] Bielecki I., Horbulewicz A., Wolan T (2012). Prevalence and risk factors for Auditory Neuropathy Spectrum Disorder in a screened newborn population at risk for hearing loss. *Int J Pediatr Otorhinolaryngol,* 76(11), 1668-1670.
[40] Sanyelbhaa Talaat H., Kabel A.H., Samy H., Elbadry M. (2009). Prevalence of auditory neuropathy (AN) among infants and young children with severe to profound hearing loss. *Int J Pediatr Otorhinolaryngol,* 73(7), 937-939.
[41] Berg A.L., Spitzer J.B., Towers H.M., Bartosiewicz C., Diamond B.E. (2005). Newborn hearing screening in the NICU: profile of failed auditory brainstem response/passed otoacoustic emission. *Pediatrics,* 116(4), 933-938.
[42] Manchaiah V.K., Zhao F., Danesh A.A., Duprey R. (2011). The genetic basis of auditory neuropathy spectrum disorder (ANSD). *Int J Pediatr Otorhinolaryngol,* 75(2), 151-158.
[43] Rapin I., Gravel J. (2003). ''Auditory neuropathy'': physiologic and pathologic evidence calls for more diagnostic specificity. *Int. J. Pediatr. Otorhinolaryngol,* 67 (7), 707–728.
[44] Berlin C.I., Morlet T., Hood L.J. (2003). Auditory neuropathy/dyssynchrony: its diagnosis and management. *Pediatr Clin North Am,* 50 (2), 331–340.
[45] Starr A., Picton T.W., Sininger Y., Hood L.J., Berlin C.I. (1996). *Auditory neuropathy. Brain,* 119, 741–753.
[46] Berlin C.I., Bordelon J., St. John P., Wilensky D., Hurley A., Kluka E., Hood L.J. (1998). Reversing click polarity may uncover auditory neuropathy in infants. *Ear Hear,* 19 (1), 37–47.
[47] Starr A., Sininger Y., Nguyen T., Michalewski H.J., Oba S., Abdala C. (2001). Cochlear receptor (microphonic and summating potentials, otoacoustic emissions) and auditory pathway (auditory brain stem potentials) activity in auditory neuropathy. *Ear Hear*, 22 (2), 91–99.
[48] Rance G. (2005). Auditory neuropathy/dys-synchrony and its perceptual consequences. *Trends in Amplification,* 9(1), 1–43.

[49] Mason J.C., De Michele A., Stevens C., Ruth R.A., Hashisaki G.T. (2003). Cochlear implantation in patients with auditory neuropathy of varied etiologies. *Laryngoscope*, 113(1), 45-49.

[50] Trautwein, P., Shallop J., Fabry, L., Friedman R. (2001). Cochlear implantation of patients with auditory neuropathy. In Y.S. Sininger and A. Starr (eds.), *Auditory Neuropathy* (pp. 203–232). San Diego: Singular Publishing.

[51] Buchman C.A., Roush P.A., Teagle H.F., Brown C.J., Zdanski C.J., Grose J.H. (2006). Auditory neuropathy characteristics in children with cochlear nerve deficiency. *Ear Hear*, 27(4), 399-408.

[52] American Academy of Pediatrics Subcommittee on Hyperbilirubinemia (2004). Management of hyperbilirubinemia in the newborn infant 35 or more weeks of gestation. *Pediatrics*, 114(1), 297-316.

INDEX

A

B

C

D

E

F

G

H

N

O

P

T

U

V

W

X